Case Studies in Psychiatry for the House Officer

Case Studies in Psychiatry for the House Officer

David A. Tomb, M.D.

*Associate Professor of Psychiatry and
Medical Director
Western Institute of Neuropsychiatry
University of Utah School of Medicine
Salt Lake City, Utah*

Daniel D. Christensen, M.D.

*Clinical Professor of Psychiatry
University of Utah School of Medicine
Salt Lake City, Utah*

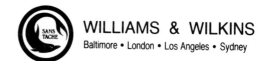

WILLIAMS & WILKINS
Baltimore • London • Los Angeles • Sydney

Editor: Kimberly Kist
Associate Editor: Linda Napora
Copy Editor: Mary Woodman
Design: JoAnne Janowiak
Production: Raymond E. Reter

Copyright © 1987
Williams & Wilkins
428 East Preston Street
Baltimore, MD 21202, U.S.A.

Accurate indications, adverse reactions, and dosage schedules for drugs are provided in this book, but it is possible that they may change. The reader is urged to review the package information data of the manufacturers of the medications mentioned.

Printed in the United States of America

Library of Congress Cataloging in Publication Data

Main entry under title:
Tomb, David A.
  Case studies in psychiatry for the house officer.
  (Case studies for the house officer)
  Includes bibliographies and index.
  1. Psychiatry—Case studies. I. Christensen, Daniel D. II. Title. III. Series.
[DNLM: 1. Mental Disorders—case studies. WM 40 T656c]
RC465.T66   1987   616.89′09   86-15812
ISBN 0-683-08339-2

86 87 88 89   10 9 8 7 6 5 4 3 2 1

Series Editor's Foreword

Case Studies for the House Officer is a series designed to teach medicine by a case-study approach. It is considered a supplement to the parent House Officer Series which provides information in a problem-oriented format. Psychiatry for the House Officer has proved very popular with house officers and medical students. In Case Studies in Psychiatry for the House Officer, Drs. Tomb and Christensen have compiled an impressive series of interesting cases that cover the most common psychiatric problems. They have done so with clarity and wit.

Lawrence P. Levitt, M.D.
Senior Consultant in Neurology
Lehigh Valley Hospital Center
Allentown, Pennsylvania
Clinical Associate Professor of Neurology
Hahnemann University and
Temple University School of Medicine

About the Authors

David A. Tomb, M.D., an adult and child psychiatrist, is an Associate Professor of Psychiatry in the Department of Psychiatry of the University of Utah School of Medicine and is the Medical Director of the Western Institute of Neuropsychiatry. He is active in teaching and in the practice of adult and child psychiatry.

Daniel D. Christensen, M.D., is the Director of Consultation-Liaison Psychiatry in the Department of Psychiatry of the University of Utah School of Medicine. He was graduated from the University of Utah School of Medicine and is active in the teaching and practice of adult psychiatry.

Preface

Patients, not textbooks, create clinicians. Even a text as well received as Psychiatry for the House Officer is only a pale reminder of the troubled individuals that provided its genesis. To bridge the gap between text and clinic, we have assembled a representative sample of cases from our practices. We will be satisfied if, through this new book, you detect a hint of the pulse of life so evident in everyday psychiatry. We will be pleased if you obtain a sense of the excitement, challenge, and pleasure of our field.

Of course, the case descriptions do not represent the whole story any more than do the questions represent all that should have been asked and the answers all that could have been said. Psychiatry, though an imperfect science, is a perfect exercise of your flexibility, creativity, and humanity. Grow with these cases; and enjoy them. Finally, let us know if you notice something that has escaped our attention - we're all in this together.

D.A.T.

D.D.C.

Acknowledgments

We wish to thank our students and residents for their enthusiasm, our colleagues for shared experiences, and our patients for educating us. Moreover, the manuscript would never have seen the light of day without the determined typing of Myrene Mandeles and Linda Miller. Nor would the book have been completed without the continuing support and encouragement of Dr. Bernard I. Grosser, Chairman of the Department of Psychiatry. Finally, we thank Dr. John H. Holbrook, Department of Internal Medicine of the University of Utah School of Medicine, for consultation on the medical aspects of several cases.

Contents

SO GOOD IT MUST BE BAD

CASE 1: A 35-year-old woman presented with the complaint
of anxiety. She was worried about her husband, the family
finances, and her marriage. On interview, her concerns
seemed justified.
    Her husband, 38-years-old, had become uncharacteristic-
ally irritable and irresponsible over the past two years.
A successful salesman of personal computers, his productivity had slackened noticeably. His moods had become increasingly unpredictable: happy and self-confident one moment,
but caustic or depressed the next hour or the next day. He
had even mentioned suicide. Recent sudden temper outbursts
caused his co-workers and his children to avoid him, yet he
could become "his old self" for days at a time.
    The family's limited savings account had been depleted
by the husband with no ready explanation. The wife had
heard rumors about an "other woman" but they remained just
rumors. Always a light social drinker, he had begun using
alcohol heavily and several times had asked his wife to
refill her prescription for diazepam (Valium). Moreover,
he had developed a keen interest in other prescription and
"street" drugs.
    If things continue unchanged, divorce seems certain.
The patient seeks help for herself yet is convinced that
the primary trouble lies with her husband.

PSYCHOBIOLOGICAL CLUE:

        Several locations in the brain are associated
    with pleasure and reward: animals with electrodes
    implanted in these areas will self-stimulate. Several
    such collections of nuclei lie in the midbrain,
    project widely to the forebrain, and are catechol-
    aminergic (primarily dopamine). Presumably, stimula-
    tion (or inhibition) of the cells in these nuclei or
    alteration of the catecholamine transmission at their
    forebrain terminals will affect mood and help create a
    sense of pleasure or despair.

QUESTIONS:

1.   Although the information above is sketchy, the husband
     probably suffers from what general type of problem?

2.   What is a likely specific etiology?

3.   Describe the acute state.

4.   Describe the chronic state.

5.   Is this disorder treatable?

1

ANSWERS:

1. Substance abuse. Although affective disorders, an
    early psychotic disorder, and an adjustment disorder
    should be considered, the rapidly fluctuating pre-
    sentation which varies from normal mood and behavior
    to that which is definitely abnormal argues against
    those possibilities and points suggestively towards
    some form of substance misuse.
        A chronic, sub-clinical medical or neurological
    illness which can cause a waxing and waning delirium
    or other organic brain syndrome should be ruled out
    (eg, porphyria, Wilson's Disease, multiple sclerosis,
    SLE). A personality disorder is ruled out by the lack
    of lifelong difficulties.

2. Cocaine abuse. The pattern of initial periods of
    enhanced self-esteem shifting over time to increased
    periods of irritability and depression is typical, as
    is faltering interpersonal relations, impaired judge-
    ment and refusal to recognize a problem, socially in-
    appropriate behavior (eg, inflated sense of sexual
    prowess with accompanying promiscuity), a tremendous
    outlay of money to buy the drug, a failing job perform-
    ance, a dissolving marriage, and increasing self-
    administration of other drugs and alcohol in an effort
    to treat uncomfortable emotional states.
        This case was unusual in the success the husband
    enjoyed in hiding his drug use from his wife (she was
    very "strict" and he knew she wouldn't approve).
    Often cocaine use is shared between husband and wife,
    or is used in fairly open social settings among
    acquaintances.

3. Cocaine is rapidly absorbed through any mucosal sur-
    face and thus is snorted (intranasal), "shot" (IV),
    smoked ("free base"), or chewed and eaten (absorption
    from buccal mucosa and GI tract).
        The goal of all this is to experience the ephem-
    eral "rush" or sense of euphoria that accompanies
    administration as well as the more prolonged (minutes
    to two hours) feelings of power, expanded capabilities,
    increased energy, alertness, and heightened self-
    esteem that follow.
        A toxic dose can progress to delusions, tactile
    hallucinations ("coke bugs"), bizarre behavior, and
    severe sympathetic discharge (tachycardia, hyper-
    pyrexia, convulsions, respiratory arrest).

4. Chronic cocaine use leads to physical dependence and
    psychological dependence.

A chronic user who stops cocaine use abruptly
will experience a mixture of symptoms (the "crash")
such as intense craving, depression, anxiety, fatigue,
insomnia, sweating and chills, and nausea and vomiting
(ie, all evidence of a physical dependence).

More intense to the chronic user is the desire to
continue using cocaine. Although their dependence is
commonly (and vigorously) denied, most serious users
seem unable to refuse the drug if it is supplied or to
stop using it until their money or supply has run out.

5.   Yes, but success is often difficult to achieve.

Severe acute intoxication can be treated with a
benzodiazepine (eg, diazepam 2.5-5.0 mg IV).

Chronic abuse is a more difficult problem and
requires a willingness to be treated. The pleasures
and sense of competence from cocaine are so profound
that, in the face of massive evidence to the contrary,
many heavy users fail to recognize their plight.
Those less involved can be treated as outpatients but
many others require hospitalization with a supportive/
confrontive peer group milieu therapy. Tricyclic
antidepressants (eg, desipramine and imipramine) may
be effective in decreasing craving and preventing
relapses.

PEARLS:

1.   More than 22 million Americans have used cocaine.

2.   The typical dose for the beginning cocaine user is
     about 50-100 mg IN, but experienced users can consume
     30 times that amount in a day.

3.   Cocaine is a CNS stimulant. Its critical effect may
     be to aid the release and block the reuptake of dopa-
     mine in the frontal lobes, but it also stimulates the
     release of norepinephrine and serotonin centrally.
     Depression may be due to the eventual depletion of
     these neurotransmitters.

4.   Cocaine administration produces arousal and persistent
     low voltage fast waves on the EEG.

5.   An intense "rush" depends on the rapid elevation of
     blood and brain cocaine levels, which in turn depends
     upon the route of administration: IN (takes 3-5 min),
     IV (14 seconds), "free-basing" (6 seconds). Thus, the
     most compelling technique is to free base, but it also
     is the most potentially addicting owing to the intense
     pleasure and reward.

6.   Some people appear predisposed to addiction by a chronic sense of inadequacy and depression which is (temporarily) relieved by cocaine use.

PITFALLS:

1.   Cocaine users are most likely to present to, and go unrecognized by, general physicians. They will not complain of cocaine use, but rather of symptoms like rhinitis and nasal sores and erosions, bronchitis, angina, hypertension, depression, and anxiety.

2.   Even the most severe of cocaine users typically insist that they are in control of the drug (a response so common as to deserve the label "cocaine delusion") - don't believe them. Cocaine may become a way of life.

3.   Death does occur with cocaine use. Severe intoxication may be fatal due to convulsions, a cardiovascular accident, or respiratory arrest. Chronic use may end in suicide.

TRIVIA:

1.   Cocaine was not deleted from "Coca-Cola" until 1906.

2.   Damage from intranasal use may result in part from the sharp microscopic crystals striking the nasal mucous membrane at speeds calculated to be as high as 120 mph.

REFERENCES

1.   Cohen S: Recent developments in the abuse of cocaine. Bull on Narcotics 36:3-14, 1984.
2.   Gawin FH, Kleber HD: Abstinence symptomatology and psychiatric diagnosis in cocaine abusers. Arch Gen Psychiat 43:107-113, 1986.
3.   Gay GR: Clinical management of acute and chronic cocaine poisoning. Ann Emer Med 11:562-72, 1982.
4.   Goeders NE, Smith JE: Cortical dopaminergic involvement in cocaine reinforcement. Science 221:773-775, 1983.
5.   Gold MS: Pharmaco-psychological effects of cocaine. Psychiatric Annals, vol 14, October, 1984.
6.   Grabowski J: Cocaine: Pharmacology, Effects, and Treatment of Abuse. NIDA Research Monograph 50, National Institute on Drug Abuse, 5600 Fishers Lane, Rockville, MD, 1984.

THE SOLITARY CYCLIST

CASE 2: A 26-year-old, recently divorced woman presented with a 5-year history of "nervousness." She has avoided crowds almost from the onset and recently any public place has become "intolerable." She is about to lose her job as a receptionist because of excessive absence and her recent refusal to attend the crowded weekly staff meeting. About three times each week she runs from her desk to the back office where she stays for about a half hour attempting to compose herself. Three years ago she became unwilling to drive on the freeway. Later she stopped driving altogether and for six months rode the bus to work. Most recently she claims, "I can't ride the bus anymore" and has begun to ride a bicycle on back roads to get to work.

At the time of symptom onset her marriage, job, and life in general were going well. She does recall that about this time she awoke at night on several occasions with a "fluttering heart" and was rushed to the emergency room fearful that she was dying. Physical and laboratory findings during these episodes were normal. Several doctors have prescribed Valium for her but with little success.

QUESTIONS:

1. What is the most likely diagnosis?

2. Name the three phases of this illness which are commonly encountered.

3. Have any biological tests proven useful in confirming the diagnosis?

4. Name three medications which have proven beneficial in treating this disorder.

5. What role does psychotherapy play in the treatment of this disorder?

ANSWERS:

1. The most likely diagnosis is Agoraphobia with Panic Attacks (DSM-III 300.21), sometimes referred to as the phobic-anxiety syndrome. "Agoraphobia," which this patient displayed, refers to symptoms such as a fear of public places and a restriction of normal life activities. The events described at the time of onset, such as "fluttering heart," fear of dying, emergency room visits, normal lab findings, and prescriptions for Valium all suggest panic attacks. In addition, it is likely that her periodic running away from her desk at work is related to ongoing panic episodes.

2. Phase I - The actual <u>panic attack</u> is usually characterized by a sudden unexplained feeling of terror accompanied by autonomic symptoms such as palpitations, dizziness, smothering, trembling, chest pains, nausea, etc.

    Phase II - <u>Anticipatory anxiety</u> often follows. Many patients become chronically anxious. This is felt to relate to their fearful anticipation that a panic attack will occur.

    Phase III - <u>Avoidance behaviors or phobias</u> often follow chronic anxiety. Presumably, the patient begins to avoid those situations which a) have been associated with a panic attack, b) they fear might precipitate a panic attack, or c) would cause embarrassment, inability to escape, or inability to reach a safe place if panic occurs.

3. Intravenous infusion of sodium lactate has been shown to precipitate panic attacks in many patients (75-85% with this disorder but not in normal controls. Following treatment with the proper medication, reinfusion of lactate usually will no longer precipitate panic.

4. Any tricyclic antidepressant can probably block panic. This was first and most convincingly shown for imipramine (Tofranil). Likewise, any MAO inhibitor will likely block panic, but this has been best documented for phenelzine (Nardil). Most recently, alprazolam (Xanax) has been proven effective in both preventing panic and controlling anticipatory anxiety. The tricyclics and MAO inhibitors usually do not directly benefit anticipatory anxiety.

5. If panic attacks are blocked with medication, some patients will rapidly lose their anticipatory anxiety and phobic avoidances. However, many will not. Educating the patient about the cause and course of the illness is often vital as is any technique (from behavior therapy to analysis) which fosters facing the avoided situations and places. Such encouragement to face the phobic situation should usually await stabilization on medication. Group therapy is no more effective than individual therapy, but in some series has appeared to bring about more rapid results.

PEARLS:

1. Panic disorder is common (about 5% of women, 1% of men). Much expensive and unnecessary testing for rare conditions (eg, pheochromocytoma) could be avoided if this condition were more often included in one's initial differential diagnosis.

2. Panic attacks do not always become complicated with anticipatory anxiety and phobic avoidances.

3. Panic disorder occurs more commonly within families. Twin studies suggest a genetic basis for this disorder.

4. Panic disorder is often associated with mitral valve prolapse (estimated as high as 50%). The significance of this finding is as yet uncertain.

5. This is a chronic remitting disorder with periods of exacerbation and remission.

6. Current neuroanatomical and psychopharmacological evidence suggests that some excessive anxiety and panic is related to overactivity of the central noradrenergic nucleus locus coeruleus, a nucleus located in the pons with projections throughout the CNS. Moreover, clonidine, an alpha-2 agonist, appears to centrally moderate both anxiety and panic attacks.

PITFALLS:

1. Valium (and other benzodiazepines) may lessen anticipatory anxiety but does not usually block panic or benefit phobic avoidances.

2. In true panic disorder, psychotherapy without proper pharmacotherapy is unlikely to be successful.

3.   Telling a patient "it's all in your head" and that he just needs to "grow up" is not helpful.

TRIVIA:

The word "panic" comes to us from the Greek shepherd god Pan. It is said that Pan would amuse himself by suddenly jumping out and frightening lonely unsuspecting travelers.

REFERENCES

1.   American Psychiatric Association Task Force on Nomenclature and Statistics: Diagnostic and Statistical Manual of Mental Disorders, 3rd ed. (DSM-III). American Psychiatric Association, Washington DC, 1980.
2.   Ballenger JC: Biology of Agoraphobia. Washington DC, American Psychiatric Press, 1984.
3.   Crowe RR, Pauls DL, Slymen DJ, et al: A Family Study of Anxiety Neurosis. Arch Gen Psychiatry 37:77-79, 1980.
4.   J Clin Psychopharmacology: 2:6, December 1982.
5.   Pauls DL, Bucher KD, Crowe RR, et al: A Genetic Study of Panic Disorder Pedigrees. Am J Hum Genet 32:639-644, 1980.
6.   Sheehan DV: Current Concepts in Psychiatry: Panic Attacks and Phobias. NEJM 307:156-158, 1982.
7.   Sheehan DV, Carr DB, Fishman SM, Walsh MM, Peltier-Saxe D: Lactate Infusion in Anxiety Research: Its Evolution and Practice. J Clin Psychiatry 46:158-165, 1985.

CASE 3: A 57-year-old chronic alcoholic was brought to the emergency room by his son. He was confused, unstable on his feet, and superficially appeared intoxicated but did not smell of alcohol. The son reported that his father "wasn't nearly this bad yesterday."

The patient had not worked in years and was living in a cold water flat off handouts and what he could borrow from his family. He ate poorly, exercised little, and drank relentlessly. Nevertheless, the family kept an eye on him and recently had become worried.

For two weeks he had been drinking little due to stomach pains. Although initially anxious and irritable, over the past several days he had become apathetic, withdrawn, and seemingly out of touch with events around him. His speech rambled, he couldn't concentrate on the TV nor remember accurately what he had seen there. He would make seemingly nonsensical statements which, however, when challenged, he could amend into something more reasonable.

Over the preceding 24 hours his condition had worsened markedly. When visited on the morning of admission, he was confused, incoherent, and so unsteady that he could not walk unaided. The son thought his father was drunk but, after inspecting the room, decided that all he had had to eat or drink was a "six-pack of Coke" (16-oz size).

In the ER he was found to be ataxic and disoriented to place and time but not to person. The physical was otherwise unremarkable. A blood alcohol level and urine drug screen were negative, and an emergency CT scan was WNL. An EEG showed diffuse slow waves but no focal events.

QUESTIONS:

1.   What is the most likely diagnosis?

2.   What "classic triad" is associated with this condition?

3.   What is the etiology of this disorder?

4.   What test will confirm the diagnosis?

5.   How is this disorder treated?

ANSWERS:

1. <u>Wernicke's Encephalopathy</u>. In our society, this condition occurs primarily in poorly nourished alcoholics.

2. <u>Ataxia</u>, <u>nystagmus</u>, and <u>confusion</u>. The complete triad occurs in fewer than half of patients.

   <u>Ataxia</u> (found in 60% of patients) results from lesions in the superior vermis of the cerebellum. In most patients additional instability is added, particularly in the acute state, by <u>impaired vestibular function</u> (positive ice-water caloric test).

   Several ocular abnormalities occur: <u>nystagmus</u> (usually horizontal; 60% of cases) due to damaged vestibular nuclei; <u>lateral rectus muscle paralysis</u> (50% of cases) due to lesions of the sixth nerve nuclei; and <u>conjugate gaze palsies</u> (40% of cases) due to third nerve nuclei lesions.

   <u>Global confusion</u> occurs in the majority of patients.

3. <u>Thiamine deficiency</u>. Although unusual, conditions of thiamine deficiency other than alcoholism may present with a typical Wernicke's encephalopathy: eg, gastric cancer, hyperemesis, extreme fasting.

   For reasons that are unclear, the <u>mammillary bodies</u> are always damaged, whereas the nuclei mentioned above are variably injured. If memory impairment is significant, there are also lesions in the <u>dorsal medial nuclei of the thalamus</u>.

4. None. No test is diagnostic; all are only suggestive. Serum thiamine levels are usually, but not invariably, low. Ultimately this is a clinical diagnosis.

5. <u>IM or IV thiamine</u> (100 mg to begin, then 50 mg daily). It is a medical emergency.

PEARLS:

1. Many cases are recognized only at autopsy, suggesting that milder, sub-clinical forms <u>may</u> be common. Did this patient have a mild form of the encephalopathy during the days prior to his sudden decompensation?

2. The ocular signs often disappear within hours of thiamine replacement, whereas the mental changes and ataxia may take weeks to improve and may never completely go away.

3. Once their confusion has lifted, 80% of "full-blown" Wernicke's patients will be found to have profound anterograde and retrograde amnesia (Korsakoff's psychosis). Only one quarter of these patients ultimately recover completely.

4. If mild forms are common, it may be possible to recognize and treat them early and thus avoid certain devastating long-term complications such as memory loss.

5. Some Wernicke's patients may have a genetic predisposition to the disease: a defect in transketolase activity (the metabolic enzyme on which thiamine acts).

6. A small percentage of patients will spend the remainder of their lives in psychiatric hospitals due to incapacitating anterograde memory loss.

7. In any confused psychiatric patient who appears poorly nourished, shoot first (with thiamine), then treat in other ways. It does no harm but can do great good.

PITFALLS:

1. If untreated until fully developed, the mortality rate among Wernicke's patients is almost 20%.

2. Carbohydrate loading in the face of poor nutrition can precipitate acute Wernicke's encephalopathy by making a sudden demand on the body's thiamine stores (eg, IV dextrose given to a starvation victim). Could a "six-pack of Coke" have precipitated this patient's acute episode?

REFERENCES

1. Blass JP, Gibson GE: Abnormality of a thiamine-requiring enzyme in patients with Wernicke-Korsakoff syndrome. NEJM 297:1367, 1977.
2. Harper C: Wernicke's encephalopathy: a more common disease than realized: A neuropathological study of 51 cases. J Neurol Neurosurg Psychiatry 42:226-31, 1979.
3. McDowell JR, LeBlanc HJ: Computed tomographic findings in Wernicke-Korsakoff syndrome. Arch Neurol 41:453-4, 1984.
4. Reuler JB, Girard DE, Cooney TG: Wernicke's Encephalopathy. NEJM 312:1035-9, 1985.
5. Victor M, Adams RD, Collins GH: The Wernicke-Korsakoff Syndrome: A Clinical and Pathological Study of 245 Patients, 82 with Post-Mortem Examinations. Philadelphia, Davis, 1971.

CASE 4: Mrs M, a 28-year-old, twice-divorced mother of 3, is hospitalized for the third time in two years after she presented to the ER complaining that she was afraid she would kill herself. For the past several days she has become increasingly despondent and tired of her life. She reports that she has made definite plans to kill herself by "slicing myself with a razor blade at every pressure point on my body."

She tells the ER intern that she wants to die because she cannot forgive her imperfections. She "messes up simple things like how she should look in the morning and whether or not she gets to work on time as well as more important things like keeping her religious vows." She notes that she is deeply religious but now is sexually active with a married man with 5 children. She wants to die because she has not only ruined her life, but his. She thinks her children would be better off without her. She describes her life as "meaningless" and says she has felt empty and lonely as long as she can remember, even when with others. She currently has no friends of either sex except the married man she is dating.

She has made many suicide attempts in the past by overdose. Moreover, she has many lacerations on her arms, chest, and abdomen (scars she seems proud of) where she has cut herself. She says the self-destructive behavior began when she was 5. She would stick herself with needles "just to watch the blood run." At 12 she took her first overdose. At 13 she claims to have watched two close friends kill themselves by slicing their abdomens open but was too scared to do it to herself. As a teenager she abused many drugs, was addicted to alcohol, "slept around" a lot, and had frequent run-ins with the police for disorderly conduct and petty theft.

She did well in high school but dropped out after one year of college to get married. She works as a hostess in a fancy restaurant, a job she has held for the past 5 years. She describes her three children as "overwhelming."

Her parents were divorced when she was 12. She fought "endlessly" with her mother and was "raped 3 times by my father." There is no family history of psychiatric illness.

During the interview and a brief mental status exam she did not appear to be particularly depressed, although she insisted that she was. She was alert, oriented, had good memory, abstracted well, denied hallucinations and delusions, and showed no evidence of thought disorder or psychosis.

Because of the specificity of her suicidal threat, she was admitted to the psychiatric unit for observation.

CLINICAL CLUE:

After reading the above report in the chart the next morning, you enter her room to meet your new patient. Before you can do more than tell her who you are, she lashes out at you with a verbal attack that questions your credentials, motivation, ethics, manhood, and lineage. She is furious - with you, with the staff, and with the hospital. You stumble from the room shaken, bewildered, and angry.

QUESTIONS:

1. What is the primary diagnosis?

2. What class of psychiatric disorders is most commonly associated with this condition?

3. Is medication of any use in this condition?

4. How would you treat this patient with psychotherapy?

5. What do you think of the psychiatrist's anger after interviewing the patient the following day?

ANSWERS:

1.   Borderline personality disorder (BPD). This patient displays many of the symptoms characteristic of BPD including self-damaging impulsivity, unstable interpersonal relationships, a sense of chronic loneliness and emptiness, substance abuse, unconventional thinking, possible dissociative episodes associated with cutting herself, and marked affective instability with anger as a prominent emotion (as the resident discovered). These patients have long-standing patterns of labile behavior often referred to as "stabile instability." Decompensation under even mild stress is common.

       Although DSM-III defines BPD by the presence of certain symptoms, many experts (primarily of psychodynamic leanings) feel that (1) symptoms are of only secondary importance, (2) the disorder is one of aberrant "personality structure," and (3) the diagnosis can only be made in the presence of a certain pattern of mental mechanisms such as splitting, denial, projection, externalization, and scapegoating. Thus, in practice, psychiatrists may use different criteria for making the diagnosis of BPD and thus may be working with different clinical populations. However, even using DSM-III standards, BPD patients probably represent an as yet unrefined spectrum of disorders rather than a single entity.

2.   Affective disorders. In fact, some experts feel that most BPD patients have subsyndromal affective disorders. Most patients at one time or another will meet the criteria for one of the affective disorders. (A review this patient's chart revealed several past diagnoses of dysthymic disorder.) In addition, so varied is their symptomatology that about half of all BPD patients will also meet the criteria for one or more additional personality disorders.

       It previously was felt that BPD was related to schizophrenia, in light of the brief confused, "psychotic" episodes that these people occasionally experience. Recent studies, however, have not confirmed that relationship; rather, schizophrenia is most likely genetically related to another condition, schizotypal personality disorder.

3.   No medication is routinely effective. A significant number of these patients, particularly but not exclusively those with prominent affective symptoms, may benefit from antidepressants. In others, lithium carbonate or low-dose antipsychotics are worth a try.

4. There is no generally accepted single way to treat
    BPD. Most experts agree that successful treatment (1)
    is usually lengthy, (2) is primarily conducted in an
    outpatient setting, (3) may occasionally require
    hospitalization during times of stress and decompensa-
    tion, and (4) may fail to provide a "cure."
        There are two prominent schools of thought. One
    argues that the fundamental personality structure must
    be changed through intensive, lengthy psychotherapy
    which focuses on the patient's chronic distortions of
    his interpersonal relationships (including that with
    the therapist). Often this is done through lengthy
    hospitalization where the patient is allowed to
    regress; at which time his more primitive response
    patterns are confronted and dealt with. The second
    viewpoint encourages a supportive, reality-oriented
    approach in which the patient adapts to environmental
    circumstances rather than regresses. Although a
    lengthy outpatient psychotherapeutic relationship is
    expected, hospitalization is kept short if possible.
    The first method aims for a cure through direct appli-
    cation of technique to the patient while the second
    method encourages improvement by insisting that the
    patient grow into a healthier state. Neither method
    has been proven superior to the other.

5. BPD patients frequently become extremely angry with
    the people around them ("borderline rage"), often with
    little or no apparent justification. It is "natural"
    to respond with anger yourself, particularly if your
    intentions were good and you feel blameless. Upon
    reflection, the psychiatrist in this case recognized
    the irrational basis for the patient's anger and was
    able to deal with her more effectively.

PEARLS:

1. BPD and affective disorders are common in the first
    degree relatives of borderline patients.

2. BPD is more common among women.

3. Only a minority of BPD patients with prominent depres-
    sive symptoms have a positive dexamethasone suppres-
    sion test (DST).

4. Difficult as BPD patients can be for their therapists,
    the problems presented to the family are often greater
    (Schulz, et al, 1985).

5.   BPD patients who abuse stimulants appear to be at an increased risk compared to normals to respond with a brief psychotic episode.

6.   Non-depressed BPD patients have the same shortened REM latencies on sleep studies as do patients with a major depression, suggesting an "affective coloring" to BPD.

PITFALLS:

1.   It is easy to overlook BPD in outpatients who present with symptoms like anxiety or depression since, in the outpatient setting, their characteristic "borderline" symptoms may be minimal.

2.   BPD patients are often exquisitely sensitive to rejection. Encouraging them to "stand on their own two feet" and "take control of their lives" may backfire as a therapeutic technique because the patient often views this as your effort to get rid of him.

3.   Be cautious that you don't respond in kind to a patient's "borderline rage" - don't let reflex anger cloud your judgment.

REFERENCES

1.   Akiskal HS, Chen SE, et al: Borderline: An adjective in search of a noun. J Clin Psychiat 46:41-48, 1985.
2.   Akiskal HS, Yerevanian BI, et al: The nosologic status of borderline personality: A clinical and polysomnographic study. Am J Psychiat 142:192-198, 1985.
3.   Andrulonis PA, Vogel NG: Comparison of borderline personality subcategories to schizophrenic and affective disorders. Brit J Psychiat 144:358-363, 1984.
4.   Baron M, Gruen R, Asnis L, Lord S: Familial transmission of schizotypal and borderline personality disorders. Am J Psychiat 142:927-933, 1985.
5.   Gordon C, Beresin E: Conflicting treatment models for the inpatient management of borderline patients. Am J Psychiat 140:979-983, 1983.
6.   Gunderson JG, Elliott GR: The interface between borderline personality disorder and affective disorder. Am J Psychiat 142:277-288, 1985.
7.   Koenigsberg HW, Kernberg OF, Schomer J: Diagnosing borderline conditions in an outpatient setting. Arch Gen Psychiat 40:49-53, 1983.
8.   Perry JC: Depression in borderline personality disorder. Am J Psychiat 142:15-21, 1985.
9.   Schulz PM, et al: The impact of borderline and schizotypal personality disorders on patients and their families. Hosp & Comm Psychiat 36:879-881, 1985.

A MEDICAL EMERGENCY

CASE 5: A previously well 23-year-old male was hospitalized because, over a two month period, he had withdrawn to
his room in response to voices which told him that his
family was attempting to poison him. Thus isolated, he ate
little and rarely cleaned himself. His physical examination
and laboratory evaluation were unremarkable except for
moderate cachexia felt to be due to self-starvation. He
received a diagnosis of Schizophreniform Disorder and was
begun on haloperidol (Haldol) 5 mg PO BID.
    His haloperidol was raised over three weeks to 10 mg
TID (30 mg daily) and his delusions began to disappear. On
day 23 a mistake was made with his medication: in addition
to his regular daily doses, he was given the full 30 mg at
bedtime as well. The next morning he was agitated,
restless, and complained of feeling "sick" although he was
afebrile. By the morning of day 25 his temperature was
38.1°C, he was diaphoretic, his blood pressure was 200/110
mm Hg, and he was increasingly anxious and agitated.
    Because he was felt to have contracted the "flu" which
then exacerbated his psychosis, his haloperidol was raised
to 40 mg daily. In spite of this medication change, his
condition worsened and by day 26 he was in and out of a
delirious state, had a temperature of 39.7°C, remained
hypertensive, and had developed a generalized muscular
hypertonicity described as "lead pipe" in nature.
    He was transferred to the ICU and listed as extremely
critical. All medications were stopped. Chest and
abdominal X-rays and a CT scan of the brain were normal.
Laboratory examinations of the blood and CSF were WNL
except for a WBC of 17,200 cells and a CPK of 582 IU
(normal range = 5-40). Over the next two days he gradually
became more obtunded and rigid.
    On the morning of day 28 his temperature was 39.5°C,
his WBC was 22,600, and his CPK was 998 IU. Later that day
he died of apparent respiratory failure.

QUESTIONS:

1. What was wrong with this man?

2. Identify the "classic tetrad."

3. Name two laboratory tests that are specifically diag-
    nostic for this condition.

4. What is the time course of this syndrome?

5. Describe the proposed biological etiology.

6. Is effective treatment available?

17

ANSWERS:

1. Neuroleptic malignant syndrome (NMS). NMS is an unusual (affects fewer than 1% of the patients at risk), unpredictable, life-threatening reaction to antipsychotic medication.

2. Hypertonicity: "lead pipe" rigidity and akinesia are common and may become severe enough to mimic catatonia.
    Hyperthermia: elevated temperature is almost invariably present and may reach as high as 40-41°C. The hyperthermia appears to be secondary to both a central disregulation and heat generated by the hypertonicity.
    Altered consciousness: agitation, anxiety, and restlessness are most common, but impairment of consciousness can progress to coma.
    Autonomic instability: a mixed pattern occurs which may include hypertension, tachycardia, dysrhythmias, and diaphoresis.

3. There are none. However, there are several consistently abnormal laboratory findings: leukocytosis (often 20,000-30,000 cells) without a left shift, elevated creatine phosphokinase, and abnormal liver enzymes.

4. NMS develops rapidly (over 1-3 days) and, even with early recognition and proper treatment, may last for weeks.

5. The patient is thought to develop a sudden hypersensitivity to the dopamine receptor blockade effect of neuroleptic drugs. Thus, the symptoms of NMS are felt to be secondary to the potentiation of the central antidopaminergic activity of these drugs, particularly in the striatum and hypothalamus.

6. Yes. The most important factor is early recognition of the syndrome and immediate discontinuation of any neuroleptics. Supportive medical care in an ICU setting may also be required.
    The most effective treatment currently available seems to be a combination of dantrolene (Dantrium) and bromocriptine mesylate (Parlodel), two drugs which work by different but synergistic mechanisms. Dantrolene is a muscle relaxant which induces a fall in body temperature and muscle destruction directly while bromocriptine is a dopamine agonist which competes with the dopamine receptor blockade centrally. Other

dopamine agonists like amantadine and levodopa have also been shown to be effective.

PEARLS:

1. The mortality rate of NMS is 20-30%. This is a dangerous condition.

2. Although anyone can be affected, younger men appear to be at particular risk as do individuals who are debilitated or physically stressed (as was the case with this cachexic patient).

3. Muscular rigidity may precede other symptoms by a day or more, so stiffness in someone taking neuroleptics should be evaluated carefully even though it is a common complaint.

4. NMS may be precipitated by a sudden increase in dosage (as probably occurred in this patient when a mistake was made with his medication).

5. NMS symptoms disappear as the neuroleptic is cleared from the body. Thus depot antipsychotics prolong recovery time.

6. Death in NMS most commonly results from respiratory failure from decreased chest wall compliance and aspiration but may also be due to cardiovascular collapse or myoglobin-induced acute renal failure.

PITFALLS:

1. Do not mistake the development of NMS in a chronic schizophrenic for the onset of catatonic schizophrenia or the worsening of the psychosis. Be guided by the presence of autonomic instability and hyperthermia.

2. NMS can occur after minimal exposure to neuroleptics (eg, after brief use as a preanesthetic medication), so don't overlook it in medical patients.

REFERENCES

1. Caroff SN: The neuroleptic malignant syndrome. J Clin Psychiatry 41:79-83, 1980.
2. Granato JE, Stern BJ, Ringel A, et al: Neuroleptic malignant syndrome: Successful treatment with dantrolene and bromocriptine. Ann Neuro 14:89-90, 1983.
3. Guze BH, Baxter LR: Neuroleptic malignant syndrome. NEJM 313:163-6, 1985.
4. Henderson VW, Wooten GF: Neuroleptic malignant syndrome: A pathogenic role for dopamine receptor blockade? Neurology 31:132-7, 1981.
5. Levenson JL: Neuroleptic malignant syndrome. Amer J Psychiat 142:1137-1145, 1985.
6. Mueller PS: Neuroleptic malignant syndrome. Psychosomatics 26:654-662, 1985.
7. Neuroleptic malignant syndrome: Lancet 1:545-6, 1984.
8. Stoudemire A, Luther JS: Neuroleptic malignant syndrome and neuroleptic-induced catatonia: Differential diagnosis and treatment. International J Psychiatry in Med 14:57-63, 1984.

CASE 6: A 30-year-old man was diagnosed as "borderline" at age 22. He had presented complaining of "bad anxiety" and an inability to relate to women. After six months of outpatient psychotherapy he made a serious suicide attempt and was hospitalized. Chlorpromazine (Thorazine) 200 mg/day was prescribed in an attempt to control future impulsive acts and settle his ongoing anxiety. On the 6th hospital day he complained of feeling stiff. He was noted to walk slowly without armswing. As he sat at rest a tremor was apparent in his right hand and forearm. These problems resolved with the addition of benztropine (Cogentin) 2 mg BID. He was discharged from the hospital after 3 weeks.

During the past 8 years he has been graduated from college and has married. Currently, both his job and marriage are sources of frustration and unhappiness. Most of his complaints revolve around boredom, depression, and marital discord. He has been hospitalized on 4 subsequent occasions, two of which followed overdoses of his medication. He has been maintained almost continuously on neuroleptics. His doctors credit the medication with preventing more serious psychotic breaks. Most recently he has been receiving fluphenazine 5 mg TID and benztropine 2 mg BID.

One month ago he began to make odd grunting sounds. He said he "couldn't help it" and often tried to divert attention from them by purposefully clearing his throat or coughing. His doctors saw this as a sign of further regression. Although the patient denied it, they speculated that he was responding to internal voices. They raised his fluphenazine dose to 30 mg/day and the noises did stop. His wife called today to complain that he has begun to walk with his back and neck bent to the right and a son reported that he heard Dad making "those same funny noises."

QUESTIONS:

1. What is the most likely diagnosis to account for the odd noises and posture?

2. What other findings would you expect to be present?

3. What is the prevalence of this disorder among those at risk?

4. What neuroleptics available in the United States are not associated with this condition?

5. How is this condition treated?

ANSWERS:

1.   Tardive dyskinesia. Tardive dyskinesia consists of
      involuntary movements which begin in conjunction with
      and are caused by neuroleptic therapy. Slow tongue
      thrusting and lip smacking are most common but tardive
      dyskinesia also includes choreoathetoid movements of
      the extremities, diaphragmatic dyscontrol (labored
      breathing, grunting, etc.), dystonias, akathisias, and
      tics. The postural component of the problem would be
      more precisely termed a tardive dystonia.

2.   You would expect the patient to also show the more
      typical orofacial or choreoathetoid movements of tar-
      dive dyskinesia.

3.   Estimates vary greatly. The most widely accepted
      figure is 15-20% of those taking neuroleptics long-
      term. Risk is increased in the aged, those with OBS,
      females, high doses of medication, simultaneous use of
      several antipsychotics, and possibly long duration of
      treatment.

4.   None. A dibenzoxazepine derivative clozapine (avail-
      able in Europe) is felt to show no or very low risk of
      tardive dyskinesia. Reserpine is felt by some to
      provide slight antipsychotic benefit without a tardive
      dyskinesia risk.

5.   Attempt to lower or discontinue the neuroleptic. If
      the offending drug is not withdrawn, the tardive dys-
      kinesia will persist. Benzodiazepines may ameliorate
      some of the abnormal movements but do not constitute
      adequate or effective treatment. Many agents are
      being investigated but none have proven useful in the
      majority of tardive dyskinesia patients. Anticholin-
      ergics are often useful in tardive dystonias but tend
      to aggravate the dyskinetic movements which are usual-
      ly also present. If total discontinuation is not ad-
      visable, the minimal dose for the minimal time should
      be employed. Switching to a different chemical class
      of neuroleptic is sometimes beneficial.

PEARLS:

1.   Tardive dyskinesia often emerges rapidly and is not
      clearly progressive.

2.   Tardive dyskinesia will commonly remit after the neuro-
      leptic is stopped, however this may take months or
      years. Some cases appear to be irreversible.

3. Both the severity and prevalence of tardive dyskinesia increase in the elderly.

4. Often the patient is unaware of early dyskinesia. A clinical rating scale for tardive dyskinesia (such as the Abnormal Involuntary Movement Scale) should be performed regularly on all patients taking neuroleptics for longer than six months.

5. A condition clinically indistinguishable from tardive dyskinesia occurs commonly in the elderly (6% of those over 60). This has been called the "spontaneous oral masticatory syndrome" and is unrelated to neuroleptic treatment.

PITFALLS:

1. Neuroleptics are too commonly prescribed for mood, character, and anxiety disorders. There is nothing in this patient's history to justify chronic neuroleptic treatment.

2. Drug-free periods (drug holidays) probably do not decrease the incidence of tardive dyskinesia. In fact, some recent data suggests that tardive dyskinesia may be more likely when chronic neuroleptic treatment includes drug holidays.

3. When tardive dyskinesia movements emerge, raising the neuroleptic dose will generally alleviate the movements. Unfortunately, this is a "masking" which only compounds the problem and creates a vicious cycle. It is only a matter of time before the involuntary movements will break through.

TRIVIA:

In 1984, 40% of malpractice suits filed against psychiatrists were related to tardive dyskinesia.

REFERENCES
1. Burke RE, et al: Tardive dystonia: Late-onset and persistent dystonia caused by antipsychotic drugs. Neurol 32:1335-1346, 1982.
2. Chiang E, et al: Respiratory dyskinesia: Review and case reports. J Clin Psychiatry 46:232-235, 1985.
3. Fahn S: A therapeutic approach to tardive dyskinesia. J Clin Psychiatry 44:19-24, 1985.
4. Jeste DV, Wyatt RJ: Prevention and management of tardive dyskinesia. J Clin Psychiatry 44:14-18, 1985.
5. Klawans HL: Recognition and diagnosis of tardive dyskinesia. J Clin Psychiatry 44:3-7, 1985.

CASE 7: Annie, a 17-year-old female, was brought by her parents to the office of their family physician. She protested the visit vigorously, insisting that there was nothing wrong and if anyone needed help it was her mom. She described bitter fights which had begun about six months ago and which centered on her choice of friends. The family discord continued at a high level and issues broadened to include her increasing neglect of friends and social activities. Her mother complained that Annie avoided the family and wouldn't even sit with them for dinner anymore. Her school work had always been excellent and, in spite of all the trouble at home, her most recent report card showed her "straight A" average to be intact.

About five months ago she began jogging five miles each morning. For Annie this took precedence over the family being together for morning breakfast. Exercise and "getting in shape" seemed to be taking more and more of her time. Moreover, her mother's complaints about Annie's nightly aerobic exercise in her room have only contributed to their strained relationship. "I can't tell her anything anymore. She is so irritable, we're thinking about having her move out."

Annie repeatedly refused any suggestion that she see the family doctor, but her parents have become more insistant as they have seen how her energy has fallen off. She is noticeably weaker and in the last week has stopped both the morning jog and the evening aerobics. They suspect that she has lost weight, but admit that they are uncertain on this point. She had previously been slightly overweight (about ten pounds), now looks thinner through the face, but is always layered in loose fitting clothes. "She's been so secretive and irritable that we wonder if she's pregnant."

At the time of her evaluation she complained of stomach pains and noted that her periods had stopped two months ago.

PHYSICAL EXAMINATION CLUES:

Pulse, 54/min and regular; temperature, 36.5°C; Blood pressure, 85/65; Height, 5'4"; Weight (6 months ago), 128 lbs.; Weight (today), 72 lbs.

LABORATORY CLUES:

Serum K^+, 2.8; EKG, "sinus bradycardia."

QUESTIONS:

1.   What is the diagnosis?

2.   What age range, sex, and social class is associated with the highest incidence of this disorder?

3.   What cultural factors are believed to be contributory?

4.   Should this patient be hospitalized?

5.   What is the most common immediate cause of death in this condition?

6.   What factors are associated with a poor prognosis?

ANSWERS:

1. <u>Anorexia Nervosa</u>. This is characterized by signifi-
    cant weight loss, disturbance of body image, intense
    fear of obesity, and refusal to maintain an appropri-
    ate body weight. Medical conditions (eg, diabetes,
    Addison's disease, tumors, etc) should be ruled out;
    however, patients with such medical conditions gener-
    ally display an appropriate concern for the weight
    loss, make efforts to regain the weight, and do not
    show body image distortion nor actively pursue thin-
    ness. Other common features this case illustrates are
    intense family discord, withdrawal from friends and
    social activities, high achievement, denial of illness,
    resistance to treatment, preoccupation with exercise,
    secretive eating behaviors, and a high level of energy
    until late in the illness. This disorder occurs in
    two main patterns. In the <u>restricting form</u>, weight
    loss is maintained by food restriction only. In the
    <u>bulimic form</u>, weight loss behavior also involves
    binges of gross overeating followed by episodes of
    self-induced vomiting.

2. Age, 14-18; Sex, female (90-95%); Social class, top
    two social levels (of five levels).

3. Idealization of thinness. Increasing pressures on
    women toward achievement.

4. Yes. Her low energy, rapid weight loss (greater than
    30% in six months), and low serum K^+ all reveal the
    severity of her condition. In addition, her evasive-
    ness, denial, and resistance suggest outpatient treat-
    ment would be unlikely to succeed.

5. Cardiac arrest.

6. Premorbid obesity, vomiting, laxative abuse, bulimia,
    and late age of onset.

PEARLS:

1. True "anorexia" is usually not present until late in
    the course of the illness. Early on, appetite is usu-
    ally increased, but firmly resisted.

2. The prevalence of anorexia nervosa is rising.

3. Amenorrhea is very common, but is not invariably
    present.

4. Current treatments are varied and include attention to general health, behavioral contracting, individual psychotherapy, and intensive family therapy. None of these treatments are certain to improve the long-term outcome. Various drug treatments have been advocated but none provides consistant benefit.

5. A recent study has shown depressive symptoms in 80% of anorexia nervosa patients. The relationship between anorexia nervosa and depression is complex and may involve a physiologic effect of starvation, an independent major depression, decreased self-esteem linked to body weight, or other factors.

6. The incidence of anorexia nervosa is greater among first degree relatives of afflicted subjects than in control relatives (6.4% of 1° relatives vs 1.3% in controls) and about half of monozygotic pairs in a recent study were concordant for anorexia nervosa. No adoption studies have been reported (aside from one isolated case report) and as yet no strong genetic case for anorexia nervosa can be made.

PITFALLS:

1. Anorexia nervosa is not simply an extreme form of dieting.

2. It is unwise to consider this disorder as "minor" or undeserving of serious medical attention. The mortality rate is 5-10%.

TRIVIA:

Anorexia nervosa was first described by Gull in 1868. Early on it was felt to be caused by pituitary insufficiency.

REFERENCES

1. American Psychiatric Association: Psychiatric Update Annual Review Volume IV, American Psychiatric Association, Washington, DC, 1985.
2. Brincat M, et al: Anorexia nervosa. Br Med J 287:1306, 1983.
3. Gershon ES, et al: Anorexia nervosa and major affective disorders associated in families: a preliminary report. In Childhood Psychopathology and Development, ed. by Guze SB, Earls FJ, Barrett JE. New York, Raven Press, 1983.
4. Halmi KH, Eckert E, LaDu TJ, Cohen J: Anorexia nervosa: treatment efficacy of cyproheptadine and amitriptyline. Arch Gen Psychiat 43:177-181, 1986.
5. Herzog DB, Copeland PM: Eating disorders. NEJM 313:295-303, 1985.
6. Hsu LKG: The treatment of anorexia nervosa. Am J Psychiat 143:573-581, 1986.
7. Nowlin NS: Anorexia nervosa in twins: Case report and review. J Clin Psychiatry 44:101-105, 1983.
8. Piran N, et al: The presence of affective disorder in patients with anorexia nervosa and bulemia. Abstract 97:133-134, presented at the 33rd Annual Meeting of the Canadian Psychiatric Association, Ottawa, September, 1983.

CASE 8: According to his parents, a 21-year-old patient was well until he received a blow to his head at age 17. Shortly thereafter he became moderately depressed, displayed a marked drop in his energy, and stopped eating. His symptoms have been unbroken and gradually worsening ever since.

During the months after the initial episode, he stopped complaining of depression and, in fact, spoke very little. He began to sleep "all the time" and appeared so lethargic that occasionally his parents had to dress him. His movements became slow and often he would stand in one place, as if lost in thought, for an hour or more. Days might pass without him speaking a word but, when frustrated, he could become angry, swear, and spit. His speech during these outbursts was often nonsensical but occasionally he made references to having great power. At other times he appeared to be responding to voices but would neither confirm nor deny those observations. Over recent weeks he has become virtually immobile and mute.

He has had numerous medical and psychiatric hospitalizations without improvement. Various medications (particularly antipsychotics) have been used for periods of up to a month without success. Because of his deteriorating course and his current incapacitation, he has been brought to the University Hospital for the "million dollar workup."

During the examination he sits silently and makes no reply to direct questions. He moves slowly and only with encouragement. A neurologic evaluation is unremarkable except that passive, forced movement of his limbs produces a sense of "waxy flexibility." If his arm is moved to an awkward position, he will leave it there for many minutes.

All laboratory tests are normal, including a CT scan and magnetic resonance imaging of the brain. The parents (and treating physician) are concerned that the patient may die due to complications from inanition and cachexia.

QUESTIONS:

1. What is the diagnosis?

2. Is the diagnosis obvious?

3. Construct a differential diagnosis.

4. Could an Amytal interview help secure the diagnosis?

5. What is the role of individual psychotherapy in this disorder?

ANSWERS:

1. Schizophrenia, Catatonic Type (DSM-III, 295.2). The crucial element here is that he first must meet the criteria for schizophrenia (bizarre delusions, auditory hallucinations, deterioration, etc) and only then is considered of catatonic type (stupor, posturing, etc).

2. No! Certainly, because of all the symptoms of catatonia, the first impulse is to conclude that the patient suffers from catatonic schizophrenia. That is always a mistake. The symptom complex known as "catatonia" is a pattern of symptoms (posturing, catalepsy, rigidity, mutism, staring, negativism, grimacing, etc) which can occur in a number of psychiatric and medical/neurological conditions and which is definitely not synonymous with catatonic schizophrenia.

   Although catatonic schizophrenia presents some positive findings like a formal thought disorder and bizarre delusions, it is essentially a diagnosis of exclusion. A spectrum of medical and psychiatric conditions must be ruled out.

3. Psychiatric disorders. Besides schizophrenia, catatonia is most commonly associated with affective, somatoform, and dissociative disorders. The occasional presence of delusions and peculiar ways of thinking in these conditions may further confuse the diagnosis.

   Neurological disorders. A host of focal (basal ganglia, limbic system, temporal lobes) and widespread (encephalitis, diffuse trauma) CNS conditions can cause the catatonic syndrome. Look for delirium, altered neurologic examination, and abnormal lab tests (eg, EEG, CSF).

   Medical disorders. Many may be responsible: particularly metabolic conditions that can produce a delirium or a stuporous state. Also common are reactions to street drugs (eg, amphetamines, PCP) and prescription medications (neuroleptics, disulfiram).

4. Yes, but not in every case. The expectation is that with IV Amytal (1) the catatonic schizophrenic will "clear" and become verbal and mobile, (2) the depressed patient will become sleepy, and (3) the medical catatonic will become more confused and/or obtunded. Unfortunately, these "classic" reactions do not always occur.

5.   Very limited. Treatment is primarily psychopharmaco-logical (antipsychotics). However, since the patients need to remain engaged in treatment and deal with reality-based issues once improvement occurs, indivi-dual therapy can provide the relationship which as-sures that this happens.

PEARLS:

1.   A common error is to mistake a catatonic state in a severely depressed individual for catatonic schizo-phrenia and thus overlook potentially effective treat-ments like antidepressant medication and ECT.

2.   Neuroleptic medication can produce both catatonic symptoms and several catatonic-like states which may be life-threatening (eg, see Case #4: the neuroleptic malignant syndrome).

3.   Catatonics <u>require</u> hospitalization; first for diagno-sis, then for treatment.

4.   The mortality rate in catatonia is high, both due to the underlying illness and to conditions like aspira-tion pneumonitis and cachexia.

5.   Always rule out encephalitis but be aware that that great mimic of psychiatric symptomatology, herpes simplex encephalitis, may have a normal spinal tap initially. Fortunately, in that condition the EEG is usually abnormal.

6.   Because these patients are occasionally completely mute, you may have to rely on family and other observers for your historical information.

PITFALLS:

1.   <u>Never</u> conclude that a patient's catatonia is psycho-genic until it has been thoroughly evaluated medically without positive findings. Even then, always keep the possibility of a medical/neurological etiology in the back of your mind.

2.   Don't assume that schizophrenia + catatonia = catatonic schizophrenia. Schizophrenics are at risk to develop medical catatonia due to poor health and chronic anti-psychotic use (ie, neuroleptic-induced catatonia).

TRIVIA:

At the turn of the century catatonic schizophrenics were extremely common and filled the mental hospitals. Today they are unusual. What has happened to them? (One thought is that many of these patients were really deteriorated depressed patients who are being effectively treated today with medication and ECT and thus don't progress to a catatonic state.)

REFERENCES

1. Abrams R, Taylor MA: Catatonia: A prospective clinical study. Arch Gen Psychiatry 33:579-581, 1976.
2. Fricchione GL: Neuroleptic catatonia and its relationship to psychogenic catatonia. Biol Psychiatry 20:304-313, 1985.
3. Gelenberg AJ: The catatonic syndrome. Lancet 1:1339-1341, 1976.
4. Kahlbaum K: Catatonia. Baltimore, Johns Hopkins Press, 1973.
5. Magrinat G, Danziger JA, Lorenzo IC, Flemenbaum A: A reassessment of catatonia. Comp Psychiatry 24: 218-228, 1983.
6. Stroudemire A: The differential diagnosis of catatonic states. Psychosomatics 23:245-252, 1982.

CASE 9: A 48-year-old janitor complains of severe daytime fatigue. He thinks it began about five years ago. "I guess I really didn't notice it at first. Now it's so bad I want to sleep all day. I can hardly do my job." He also complains of depression and pounding headaches. By his wife's report he is very irritable. "He seems depressed to me too. On his days off he just lies around and complains that he is too tired to do anything." She adds that their marriage seems to be breaking up. "I can't stand to sleep in the same room with him at night. He snores so loud the neighbors can hear. He used to wake me up every night by making gasping noises. At first I was really scared, but now I just sleep downstairs."

On physical examination, he presents as an unshaven, moderately obese, depressed-looking man. BP = 145/105; pulse = 85/min and regular.

QUESTIONS:

1. What is the diagnosis?

2. Name four key characteristics of the "typical" patient.

3. What is the pathophysiology of this disorder?

4. Are any medical complications associated with this problem?

5. What mental/emotional complaints are common among these patients?

ANSWERS:

1. <u>Sleep Apnea</u> increasingly has been recognized as a frequent cause of daytime hypersomnia, lethargy, and sleepiness. In this syndrome respiratory compromise, apnea, or central hypoventilation at night leads to repeated interruptions of sleep. Oxygen saturation falls sufficiently to evoke recurrent, brief nighttime awakenings and cause some degree of cerebral anoxia. These events are felt to underly the common daytime complaints.

2. Middle-age, male, overweight, loud snorer.

3. The most commonly identified pathophysiology is a structural impairment of the nasopharyngeal airway. However, a few cases seem to be "central apneas": ie, caused by CNS abnormalities which reduce the drive to breathe.

4. Yes. Arrhythmias, heart failure (cor pulmonale), pulmonary hypertension, systemic hypertension, and sinus arrest.

5. Depression, irritability, memory impairment, inattention, impotence, and lethargy.

PEARLS:

1. Some people have speculated that sleep apnea is the cause of the sudden infant death syndrome.

2. Patients with sleep apnea are often unaware of sleep interruptions or respiratory problems.

3. In normal subjects, sleep is accompanied by decreased respiratory function (decreased rate, minute ventilation, respiratory drive to hypercapnia, mucociliary clearance, and smooth and intercostal muscle tone).

4. Snoring - usually loud and intermittent - is almost invariably present in the obstructive form. The pauses in snoring correspond to the apneic episodes. In REM sleep, apneic periods are longer and oxygen saturation falls lower than in non-REM sleep.

5. Sleep apnea in a thin individual is often accompanied by upper airway pathology such as a large uvula, large tongue, palatal webbing, or large tonsils.

6. Sleep apnea may occur in children. However, behavior problems rather than daytime somnolence is more often

the presenting complaint.

7. Treatment must address the underlying pathology and may involve tonsillectomy, nasal septal reconstruction, tracheostomy, decongestants, tricyclic antidepressants, or respiratory stimulants.

PITFALLS:

1. A complaint of insomnia does not rule out this disorder. Some sleep apnea patients present with the complaint of disturbed nighttime sleep. Also, some who are aware of their sleep apnea have insomnia related to a fear of the jeopardy that sleep presents for them.

2. The diagnosis is rarely made without information from the patient's family or bed partner. They usually report continuous brief arousals following what sounds like choking or gasping for air.

3. Sleep apnea is not a rare disorder. Such patients constitute one of the major groups of patients seen at sleep disorder centers.

4. Hypnotics may be dangerous to these patients.

TRIVIA:

Some sleep apnea patients have been observed to have as many as one thousand apneic episodes in a single night.

REFERENCES

1. Bixler EO, Kales A, Saldazos CR, et al: Sleep apneic activity in a normal population. Res Commun Chem Pathol Pharmacol 36:141-152, 1982.
2. Gerriss G: Sleep Disorders. Neurologic Clinics 2:51-69, 1984.
3. Frank Y, Krauath RE, Pollock CP, et al: Obstructive sleep apnea and its therapy: Clinical and polysomnigraphic manifestations. Pediatrics 71:737-742, 1983.
4. Kwentus J, Schulz SC, et al: Sleep apnea: A review. Psychosomatics 26:713-724, 1985.
5. Mendelson WB, Garnett D, Gillan JC: Flurazepam-induced sleep apnea syndrome in a patient with insomnia and mild sleep-related respiratory changes. J Nerv Ment Dis 169:261-264, 1981.
6. Zorick F, Roehrs T, et al: Patterns of sleepiness in various disorders of excessive daytime somnolence. Sleep 5:S165-S175, 1982.

CASE 10: A 56-year-old male is brought to the emergency room by his wife. She complains that he has been "losing his mind" for a long time but has been noticeably worse since yesterday. By her reports, he had had no real trouble until about six years ago. At that time he awoke one morning feeling weak and said that his right leg had "fallen asleep." He refused his wife's suggestion to see a doctor and, as he predicted, the symptoms went away. Over the following three years he experienced several bouts of depression and occasionally complained that he could no longer work hard at the job. Moreover, his business partners had recently suggested that he was beginning to make poor investments.

After an outstanding college career he had built a successful business which employed four hundred workers. He was known for his stern manner, good business sense, long hours of work, and stubborn insistence that things be done his way. In his infrequent physical examinations he had always been healthy except for mild obesity, high blood pressure, and a "smoker's cough." Doctors had advised him to lose weight, stop smoking, and take a "blood pressure pill" but he had no time for such nonsense and repeatedly told them to give their pills to someone who was sick.

He continued to work until about one year ago. Casual acquaintances noticed little but his wife and close associates often commented that they could no longer trust his judgment. His wife described that every several months she would begin to get used to how he was and "all of a sudden he'd get worse."

In the emergency room he presented in an uncooperative and irascible manner. He refused to answer any questions but commented that this was the worst hotel he had ever stayed in.

PHYSICAL EXAMINATION CLUES:

BP - 190/140; pulse - 190/min and regular; weakness was present in the right arm; deep tendon reflexes were obviously asymmetric.

QUESTIONS:

1. What is the most probable diagnosis to account for his mental condition?

2. What historical findings are commonly associated with this diagnosis?

3. What physical findings are commonly associated with this diagnosis?

4. Would an EEG be helpful in making the diagnosis?

5. What is the usual course of this illness?

6. What is the prognosis?

7. What premorbid personality features are present and what role did they play in this illness?

ANSWERS:

1. <u>Multi-infarct Dementia</u>. This term implies a loss of intellect resulting from infarction of brain tissue. Vascular disease (atherosclerosis) is the presumed underlying cause. Multi-infarct dementia results from numerous strokes (large or small) over time. A single stroke does not generally cause dementia.

2. Abrupt onset, stepwise deterioration, fluctuating course, nocturnal confusion, previous strokes, and a history of hypertension.

3. Hypertension, focal neurologic signs (eg, positive Babinski, focal weakness, asymmetric reflexes, and dysarthria), and indications of atherosclerosis (eg, funduscopic abnormalities, carotid bruit, and evidence of an enlarged heart).

4. No. EEG findings are either normal or unpredictably abnormal. However, the CT scan usually shows multiple areas of decreased density (infarction).

5. Abrupt onset with a stepwise course characterized by alternating periods of relative stability and rapid deterioration. The episodes of deterioration are felt to coincide with new infarctions. This is in contrast to the more uniformly progressive course of Alzheimer-type dementia.

6. The prognosis in multi-infarct dementia is poor in spite of active treatment. Most such patients are dead within four years of the diagnosis.

7. The premorbid personality characteristics represented in this case are primarily compulsive in nature (eg, excessive devotion to work, stubbornness, driven ambition, and the need to control people, events, and emotions). Such people are often time pressured, tense, and unable to relax - all factors which have been associated with the development of hypertension. Also, his arrogant denial prevented appropriate early treatment which might have slowed or even prevented the devastating outcome.

PEARLS:

1. Multi-infarct dementia is common, accounting for about 20% of dementias in the elderly. Only Alzheimer-type dementia, which accounts for about 50%, is more common.

2. Multi-infarct dementia and Alzheimer-type dementia can coexist. This has been called "mixed dementia."

3. Multi-infarct dementia may be associated with potentially reversible conditions such as hypertension and recurrent emboli from the heart or carotid arteries. Appropriate treatment may arrest further deterioration, slow progression, or even allow for some recovery.

4. Depression and relative preservation of the personality are rare in Alzheimer-type dementia yet occur frequently in multi-infarct dementia.

5. Signs and symptoms shown in multi-infarct dementia are a function of the brain regions which have been infarcted and are therefore "patchy." Some cognitive functions may remain intact while others show marked deterioration.

PITFALLS:

1. Aging per se does not cause dementia.

2. Some professionals still assume that the diagnosis of dementia implies irreversibility. Since the advent of DSM-III nomenclature, "dementia" refers only to clinical symptoms and carries no prognostic implications. Reversibility is a function of the underlying pathology and the application of timely, appropriate treatment.

TRIVIA:

The earliest recorded case of an infarct-type dementia is that which occurred in the famous anatomist and physician, Marcello Malpighi (about 1694). He suffered a stroke. With treatment (bleeding and powdering his feet) Dr. Malpighi recovered motor function, but was left with emotional lability, impaired memory, and poor judgment.

REFERENCES

1. Bucht G: Dementia of the Alzheimer type and multi-infarct dementia. J Amer Geriatr Soc 32:491-498, 1984.
2. Liston EH, LaBue A: Clinical differentiation of primary degenerative and multi-infarct dementia: A critical review of the evidence. Biol Psychiatry 18:1451-1465, 1983.
3. Read SL, Jarvik LF: Cerebrovascular disease in the differential diagnosis of dementia. Psychiatric Annals 14:100-108, 1984.

MYSTERIOUS MARCI

<u>CASE 11:</u> Marci, 16 years old, was taken to the office of a
psychologist by her mother. She complained that ever since
she and her alcoholic husband had separated six months
before, her daughter had been "out of control." About this
time, Marci was caught shoplifting earrings from a neighborhood convenience store. She had no explanation for her
actions beyond, "I just liked them and wanted them. So I
took them." In subsequent weeks Marci looked depressed.
She would cry at the slightest provocation and complained
of feeling ugly and fat. Then she began to lock herself in
her bedroom each evening after her typically small dinner
and would not let anyone in. Even friends or phone calls
would not cause her to come out. In the morning she would
leave for school without breakfast, saying little to her
mother or younger sister. A worried schoolmate called in
confidence, reporting that she had seen Marci smoking
marijuana at lunch time. Her mother had wondered if the
"problem was drugs" and searched Marci's room for clues.
She later reported, "Nothing seemed out of the ordinary
except for some cigarettes. I didn't know she had started
smoking. Also, I couldn't believe the mess under her bed,
but you know teenage girls. There must have been twenty
old doughnut boxes and those candy wrappers probably go
back for years."

When Marci complained of always being tired and of
having stomach aches, she was taken to her family
physician. He found a low serum potassium (3.2 meq/l) and
a mildly elevated BUN (25 mg%), swollen but painless
parotid glands, and an unusual scarring and callus
formation on the dorsum of the second and third fingers of
her right hand. He suggested she begin eating breakfast
and not worry so much about her weight. After all, 115 lbs
was "just right" for her height of 5'3". On his
suggestion, Marci was taken to the psychologist. There she
was counseled for a few weeks about accepting her parents'
separation. The correct diagnosis was finally made by a
dentist during Marci's annual check-up.

QUESTIONS:

1. What is the most likely diagnosis?

2. What is the dentist likely to have seen that led him
    to the correct diagnosis?

3. What was the cause of the scarred, callous skin on the
    dorsum of her right hand?

4. This problem has been compared to alcoholism.   What
    features do these disorders have in common?

5. What cultural factors seem to contribute to the inci-
    dence of this disorder?

6. What two groups of medications have been used with
    some success in the treatment of this disorder?

ANSWERS:

1. __Bulimia.__ Bulimia is a disorder characterized by an abnormal eating pattern consisting of binge eating alternating with little or no food intake. The binges are usually done in secret and involve easily ingested food. They often are followed by purging and feelings of depression and guilt. Other common features of bulimia which this case illustrates are precipitation by a stressful event (often a loss or separation), secretive binges occurring during evening and nighttime hours, concurrent impulsiveness in other areas such as stealing and drugs, depression, concern about body weight, complaints of lethargy and abdominal pain, hypokalemia (secondary to vomiting), increased BUN (secondary to dehydration), painless swelling of the parotid glands, and a family history of alcoholism.

2. It is not unusual for a dentist to make the diagnosis of bulimia first. He probably saw decalcification of the lingual, palatal, and posterior occlusive surfaces of the teeth. The erosion takes a pattern of rounded contours without staining and is secondary to the acid from repeated vomiting.

3. This finding occurs in bulimics who induce vomiting using their fingers to stimulate emesis. The dorsum of the fingers and hand repeatedly rub against the teeth resulting in callus formation.

4. Loss of control over the use of the substance, intense preoccupation with the substance, secretive use, and social isolation are common to both disorders. Studies have shown a family history of alcoholism is present in as many as 1/3 of bulimic patients. Perhaps patients at risk for one substance abuse pattern (drugs, alcohol, or food) may be at higher risk for another. MMPI studies have shown similarities in the profiles of bulimic, alcoholic, and drug abusing women.

5. A premium on thinness and an abundance of food.

6. __Anticonvulsants__ were first suggested when EEG abnormalities were reported in a group of bulimic patients. Some patients do respond to phenytoin with fewer binges but many do not.

   __Antidepressants__ appear to be effective in many bulimics, particularly when affective symptoms are present.

PEARLS:

1. Food consumed during a bulimic binge is usually eaten
    in a driven, rapid manner with no real enjoyment.

2. As a rule, bulimics know that their eating pattern is
    abnormal and feel a troublesome sense of loss of con-
    trol.

3. An eating binge will often continue until abdominal
    pain begins, someone discovers or interrupts it,
    sleep ensues, or vomiting is induced.

4. Studies show binge eating to be very common in college
    age women (over 50%). Rigid criteria selecting those
    in whom bulimia is present as a significant eating
    disorder shows a prevalence of about 1%.

5. Bulimia occurs mostly in women (about 95%).

6. As a rule, bulimic patients do not eat normally even
    between binges. Fasting for prolonged periods, hoard-
    ing food, and eating only certain foods are common.

7. Family studies show a higher prevalence of depression
    and alcoholism in the families of bulimic patients.

8. Bulimics may employ a variety of techniques to prevent
    weight gain. These include vomiting, laxatives, diet
    pills, enemas, and spitting out the food before it is
    swallowed.

9. Most individuals with bulimia are within the normal
    weight range. Weight fluctuations are virtually never
    so extreme as to be life-threatening.

PITFALLS:

1. Not asking about bulimic behavior during examinations
    contributes to the usual 5-7 year delay between initial
    symptoms and treatment.

2. Anorexia nervosa and bulimia are not unrelated disor-
    ders. The two occur together more than 50% of the
    time.

TRIVIA:

1. Bulimic patients can consume as many as 50,000 calor-
    ies in one binge.

2. Bulimic habits may cost the patient more than $20-30 a day. Like drug addicts, some resort to stealing to support their habit.

REFERENCES

1. American Psychiatric Association Task Force on Nomenclature and Statistics: Diagnostic and Statistical Manual of Mental Disorders, 3rd ed. (DSM-III). Amer Psychiatric Association, Washington, DC, 1980.
2. American Psychiatric Association: Psychiatric Update Annual Review Volume IV, American Psychiatric Association, Washington, DC, 1985.
3. Brotman AW, Herzog AB, Woods SW: Antidepressant treatment of bulimia: The relationship between binging and depressive symptomatology. J Clin Psychiatry 45:7-9, 1984.
4. Hatsukami D, Owen R, Pyle R, et al: Similarities and differences on the MMPI between women with bulimia and women with alcohol and drug abuse problems. Addictive Behaviors 7:435-439, 1982.
5. Herzog, DB: Bulimia: The secretive syndrome. Psychosomatics 23:481-487, 1982.
6. Hughes PL, Wells LA, Cunningham CJ, Ilstrup DM: Treating bulimia with desipramine. Arch Gen Psychiat 43:182-186, 1986.

CASE 12: A 22-year-old male was taken to a psychiatrist by his concerned parents. They complained that he had no interest in girls and dating and had just been fired from his third job this year. They feared that he would never leave home. They said he had always been "a little different."

The pregnancy was complicated by toxemia and a hard delivery. At fourteen months of age he was hospitalized with a high fever and seizures. In school he was often accused by the teacher of not paying attention and even his parents thought he was a daydreamer. They added that he also has had "spells" in which he has seemed dizzy, looked over to one side, and chewed. Moreover, these occasional spells continue at the present time. He did poorly in high school, went on few dates, and has never seemed to have any real interest in girls. His parents described him as serious, very religious, and often angry.

The patient presented in a stern, humorless manner. He was dressed and groomed appropriately but his speech was intense and circumstantial and included many details, clarifications, and qualifications. In addition, he presented a 38-page "summary" describing the few dates he had been on. In passing, he commented that in the last two months he had filled seven spiral notebooks with his writings. He had no complaints about dating or girls, saying he just wasn't interested in anything serious. On further questioning, it was apparent that he lacked sexual interest, had no sexual dreams or fantasies, and had never experienced an orgasm. No delusions or hallucinations were present, yet he manifested an extreme preoccupation with religious, moral, and philosophical issues. When the consultation hour was up, the patient continued to talk and resist the doctor's efforts to terminate the interview. In the following week he called the office twice to expand on issues and sent three lengthy letters.

A physical examination showed no abnormalities. Secondary sexual characteristics were normally developed. A neurologic exam, routine laboratory data, EEG, and CT scan were all within normal limits.

QUESTIONS:

1. What is the diagnosis?

2. What common features of this disorder does this case illustrate?

3. What common features of this disorder are not presented by this case?

4. Why is the EEG normal?

45

ANSWERS:

1. Temporal Lobe Epilepsy, now often referred to as par-
    tial complex seizures. The various symptoms of
    temporal lobe epilepsy can be conceptualized as fall-
    ing into five areas:
    1. Preictal symptoms such as lethargy, dizziness,
        irritability, or ataxia.
    2. Aura symptoms such as epigastric sensations;
        various emotions; time, auditory, or visual
        distortions; and olfactory or gustatory sen-
        sations.
    3. The ictus, usually consisting of simple or
        complex automatisms and alterations of con-
        sciousness.
    4. Postictal symptoms such as confusion, amnesia,
        aphasia, and fatigue.
    5. Interictal symptoms such as hypergraphia,
        altered sexual behavior, intense emotions,
        and interpersonal clinging. (These have
        been referred to as the "interictal behavior
        syndrome.")

2. Pre- and perinatal complications, childhood febrile
    seizures, hyposexuality, being perceived as a day-
    dreamer, stern humorless demeanor, hypergraphia, cir-
    cumstantial speech, anger, interpersonal clinging,
    automatisms, lapses in consciousness, and excessive
    religious/philosophical concerns.

3. Sexual deviation, overt aggression, extremes of mood,
    fears, paranoia, delusions, hallucinations, illusions,
    dissociative states, and auras.

4. A standard "awake" EEG (scalp electrodes only) fails
    to detect a deep temporal lobe focus in about half of
    patients. Diagnostic sensitivity is enhanced by sleep
    deprivation and sphenoidal or nasopharyngeal recording
    electrodes.

PEARLS:

1. Temporal lobe epilepsy is a common illness. It is the
    most frequent form of epilepsy in adults (0.3%
    prevalence).

2. It is estimated that 30-40% of temporal lobe epilepsy
    patients experience psychiatric symptoms.

3. Aggression and violence are much more common as
    interictal events than as part of the actual seizure.

4. In a recent study, aggressive temporal lobe epileptics were distinguished from aggressive character disorders by the presence of bizarre humor, philosophical interests, religiosity, circumstantiality, and interpersonal clinging.

5. Hamartomas and hippocampal sclerosis are the most commonly identified pathologic etiologies. The frequency of these lesions is felt to increase with pre- and perinatal injuries, prolonged febrile seizures, and trauma to the base of the skull.

6. Much of the aberrant thought and behavior associated with temporal lobe epilepsy is interictal.

7. Hyposexuality is most likely to be present and feel "natural" when temporal lobe epileptiform discharge is present prior to puberty.

PITFALLS:

A physician unfamiliar with the symptoms and presentation of temporal lobe epilepsy will often misdiagnose the problem as schizophrenia. All of the core schizophrenia symptoms have been reported in temporal lobe epilepsy. In contrast to schizophrenia, however, the epileptic patients generally have appropriate affects and no deterioration over time.

TRIVIA:

1. In 1979, epilepsy was cited as a defense in five U.S. murder trials.

2. Early investigators concluded that seizures and psychosis were antagonistic. This erroneous observation led Von Meduna to his early experiments with convulsive treatments for schizophrenia.

REFERENCES

1. American Psychiatric Association: <u>Psychiatric Update Annual Review Volume IV</u>, American Psychiatric Association, Washington, DC, 1985.
2. Bear DM, Freeman L, Greenberg M: Behavioral alterations in patients with temporal lobe epilepsy. In <u>Psychiatric Aspects of Epilepsy</u>, ed. by Blunes D, Washington, DC, American Psychiatric Press, 1984.
3. Gevinsky O, Bear DM: Varieties of aggressive behavior in patients with temporal lobe epilepsy. Amer J Psychiatry 141:651-655, 1984.
4. Theodore WH, Porter RJ, Perry KJ: Complex partial seizures: Clinical characteristics in differential diagnosis. Neurology 33:115-121, 1983.
5. Waxman SA, Geschwind N: The interictal behavior syndrome of temporal lobe epilepsy. Arch Gen Psychiatry 32:1580-1586, 1975.

A CASE OF IDENTITY

CASE 13: A 58-year-old, white male is brought into the emergency room by his wife and son. He was working as an architect and doing well until three weeks ago. At that time, he became noticeably more quiet and began to withdraw to his room immediately after dinner. One week ago he refused to go to work, stopped eating, and began to pace the floor at night. He would wring his hands, clench his fists, and cry. He talked of many minor life events as being "major sins" and today began to warn his family that he was really "the devil." "All these years you've mistaken me for your father. I am the devil, Satan himself. No one is more evil and wretched than me. I bring death and disease to the world and I will burn in Hell forever." This is the third time in five years he has presented in such a state. Each time he has professed the belief that his identity has been mistaken and he is really the devil.

QUESTIONS:

All features of this presentation are consistent with the DSM-III diagnosis of major depression, recurrent, with mood-congruent psychotic features (DSM-III 296.22).

1. Name two other diagnostic terms that could be used to describe this condition.

You choose to hospitalize the patient and treat with haloperidol (up to 10 mg PO QID).

2. What therapeutic response would be most likely?

You choose to hospitalize the patient and treat with imipramine (up to 300 mg/day).

3. What therapeutic response would be most likely?

You choose to hospitalize the patient and treat with a combination of amitriptyline (up to 200 mg/day) and perphenazine (up to 48 mg/day).

4. What therapeutic response would be most likely?

After six weeks of inpatient treatment with amitriptyline (250 mg/day) and perphenazine (48 mg/day) the patient has shown no appreciable response. Blood levels indicate that both medications are well within the therapeutic range.

5. What would you next recommend?

ANSWERS:

1. The terms "psychotic depression" and "involutional melancholia" date back many years but are still used by some professionals to identify this condition. Others might use the term "delusional depression" or "delusional unipolar depression". All of these terms refer to a severe depression, usually characterized by marked functional impairment, high suicide risk, the need for hospitalization, and impaired reality testing. For brevity, the term "psychotic depression" will be used in the discussion of this case.

2. Neuroleptics alone will benefit such symptoms as insomnia, anxiety, agitation, and delusional thinking but do not benefit the core depressive symptoms. For this reason, neuroleptic medication alone is generally ineffective in the treatment of psychotic depression and would be a poor choice in this case. (Loxapine may be an exception to this rule. An active metabolite of loxapine is the antidepressant amoxapine).

3. Early studies indicated that antidepressants alone (both tricyclic antidepressants and MAO inhibitors) were ineffective treatment for psychotic depression. More recent studies involving high doses and plasma level monitoring have reconfirmed this observation. In this case, antidepressants alone would be a poor therapeutic choice. (Amoxapine, having known neuroleptic/dopamine antagonistic activity, may be an exception).

4. Combined neuroleptic-antidepressant therapy is the most effective pharmacological treatment for psychotic depression. The amitriptyline-perphenazine combination is commonly prescribed and well studied. Some contend that the two preparations should be administered separately with the antipsychotic begun first. This may (1) protect against exacerbation of the psychosis by the antidepressant, (2) more rapidly lessen agitation and anxiety, (3) allow for more accurate assessment of side effects, and (4) allow the antipsychotic to be stopped while continuing the antidepressant.

   Others advocate a fixed combination preparation (Triavil or Etrafon) claiming (1) better patient compliance because of fewer pills, (2) decreased risk of acute extrapyramidal symptoms because of the anticholinergic effect of the antidepressant, and (3) a decreased risk of tardive dyskinesia. Whether any of these arguments are correct is as yet unproven.

5. The best choice at this point would be electroconvul-
    sive therapy (ECT). Some clinicians would have begun
    directly with ECT treatment and a small number of
    others would likely have begun with combined ECT-
    antidepressant therapy. However, the most widely
    accepted practice is to provide an adequate trial of
    medication, followed by ECT if the response is in-
    adequate.
        Since the initial comparison studies in 1964, ECT
    has been generally accepted as more effective and
    safer than any antidepressant, antipsychotic, or
    tricyclic-antipsychotic combination in the treatment
    of psychotic depression. Thus, the common habit of
    beginning treatment with medication - neither the
    safest nor the most humane practice - probably is a
    reflection of the conservative posture with which most
    practitioners prescribe ECT.

PEARLS:

1. Psychotic depression is almost always recurrent and is
    felt to be endogenous (ie, biological).

2. Psychotic depression is more common in women than men
    (about 2:1).

3. Psychotic depression is uncommon in young adults and
    occurs more frequently with increasing age.

4. The incidence of psychotic depression is rising - prob-
    ably related to the increasing number of elderly indi-
    viduals in the population.

5. As a rule, the delusional content in psychotic depres-
    sion is similar from episode to episode.

PITFALLS:

1. Psychotic depression is, as a rule, unresponsive to
    psychotherapy or hospitalization alone. Effective
    treatment requires proper medication or ECT.

2. Neuroleptics prescribed for psychotic depression should
    be discontinued as soon as possible. Maintenance
    neuroleptic treatment in psychotic depression is not
    necessary and recent evidence indicates that individ-
    uals with affective disorders may be at increased risk
    for developing tardive dyskinesia.

REFERENCES

1. Anton RF, Sexauer JD: Efficacy of amoxapine in psychotic depression. Am J Psychiatry 140:1344-1347, 1983.
2. Ayd FJ: Pharmacotherapy for psychotic depression. Psychiatric Annals 8:506-507, 1985.
3. Clower CG: Recurrent psychotic unipolar depression. J Clin Psychiatry 44:216-218, 1983.
4. Glassman AH, Rouse SP: Delusional depression. Arch Gen Psychiatry 38:424-427, 1981.
5. Magure C, Nelson JC, Price LH: Reliability and validity of the symptoms of major depressive illness. Arch Gen Psychiat 43:451-456, 1986.
6. Perry PJ, Morgan DE, Smith RE, Tsuang MT: Treatment of unipolar depression accompanied by delusions. J Affect Dis 4:195-200, 1982.

CASE 14: H.M.S., a 19-year-old single male, was brought by police to the emergency room after he had been found standing in a busy intersection directing traffic. He expressed in a loud voice how signals from his mind were controlling all automobiles. It was found that he had been riding a bus cross-country when his ceaseless loud talk and bawdy sexual invitations to both men and women resulted in his being forced off the bus by the driver and several irate passengers. In the ER he refused to sit or lie down and bragged repeatedly about his energy, strength, and "mind powers." His speech was loud and incessant. Attempts to interrupt him were met by angry threats. He made little sense, jumped from one topic to another, and often laughed in a loud, inappropriate manner.

The police made contact with his parents in a neighboring state. They reported no prior history of psychiatric trouble and no known drug abuse. His mother reported that about eight days ago he began boasting and becoming aggressive in a manner very unlike his usual gentle nature. They worried further when they noticed that he was sleeping and eating very little. Five days ago, he rudely grabbed $120 from his mother as she was leaving to shop, shouted that he was going to start "the world's biggest business," ran out of the house, and had not been seen since. His mother reported that her grandfather and two uncles all had "schizophrenic episodes where they would go crazy and then come back to normal." A cousin and a daughter from the mother's first marriage (H.M.S.'s half-sister) had committed suicide.

By history and presentation, the diagnosis appeared to be Bipolar Disorder, manic, with psychotic features (DSM-III, 296.44).

QUESTIONS:

1. Should any other diagnostic possibilities be considered?

2. Could this patient be treated as an outpatient?

3. What are the chances that this person, if left untreated, would experience a severe depression at some point in his life?

4. Are there any advantages to having this disorder?

5. What treatment would you prescribe?

ANSWERS:

1.   Mania occurs most commonly as a phase of bipolar disorder, but can also result from drugs (stimulants,
steroids, L-Dopa, etc), medical conditions (tertiary
syphilis, thyrotoxicosis, systemic lupus erythematosus,
multiple sclerosis, infections, etc), sleep depriva-
tion, following child delivery ("postpartum mania"),
and extreme psychological stress (such as manic grief
reactions). In addition, paranoid schizophrenia with
grandiose delusions should be considered as a diagnostic possibility.

2.   Probably not. His release would be unwise and risky.
Civil commitment should be instituted if necessary.
Hospitalization is almost always necessary to protect
the acute manic from severe physical, social, sexual,
financial, and legal consequences. Such patients are
commonly dangerous to themselves and others, lack
insight into their delusional thinking, lack awareness
of the dangers they create, and generally have no
reason for participating in treatment. Some hypomanic
episodes or minor relapses can be treated without
hospitalization provided the patient is cooperative
and the family supportive.

3.   The chances are high. Unipolar mania (a lifetime of
recurrent mania without any depressive episodes)
occurs, but is very rare. About 80% of patients who
have an initial manic episode will have subsequent
manic and/or depressive episodes.

4.   Disadvantages to having bipolar disorder far outweigh
any advantages, yet some positive elements can, exist.
Those with a prominent hypomanic temperament are often
energetic, ambitious, creative, and driven, and attain
some social success and positions of leadership. Several studies show an association between bipolar
illness and upper social class, and bipolar women tend
to marry into higher social classes. The more serious
disadvantages include those obviously associated with
psychotic episodes and paralyzing depressions, as well
as substance abuse, divorce, and suicide. Fifteen
percent of the affectively ill commit suicide, compared
with 0.01% of the general population.

5.   The benefit of lithium therapy in acute mania has been
documented in over 100 publications, involving over
3,000 patients, in 20 countries. Statistically, about
80% of patients respond within three weeks. For more
rapid control of manic symptoms, it is common practice

to combine an antipsychotic with the lithium until the patient is stable. For patients unresponsive to or intolerant of lithium, carbamazepine may be an effective alternative.

Used prophylactically, lithium is effective in the prevention of relapses.

PEARLS:

1. Onset is most commonly during the 20's. Manic and hypomanic episodes are rare, but not unknown, before puberty. Likewise, a first episode of mania after age 65 is unusual.

2. When psychotic symptoms occur in affective illness, they are characteristically present at the height of the mania or depth of the depression. When such psychotic symptoms persist beyond the affective syndrome, a schizoaffective diagnosis becomes more likely.

3. Decreased need for sleep and an increase in activity level are among the most reliable indicators of mania.

4. If left untreated, the average female with the onset of bipolar disorder at age 25 would be expected to lose 14 years of productivity (work, school, or household responsibilities) and 9 years of life.

5. About 12% of bipolar patients stop cycling after age 65.

6. The lifetime risk for bipolar disorder is 1.2%, making it slightly more common than schizophrenia.

7. The term "Bipolar II" has been used to designate those patients with depressions and hypomania. This is a common condition accounting for about 50% of bipolar patients. The term "Unipolar II" has been used for those with recurrent depressions but a bipolar family history.

PITFALLS:

1. Misdiagnosis of bipolar illness as schizophrenia has led to large malpractice judgments when improperly used neuroleptics resulted in tardive dyskinesia. Do not be fooled by mood-incongruent delusions and hallucinations. These are not uncommon in mania. Schneider's "firsk rank symptoms," previously considered pathognomonic for schizophrenia, may occur in as many as 25% of manic-depressives.

2.   Patients with an affective disorder may be at increased risk of developing tardive dyskinesia.

3.   Depressed bipolar patients can switch into mania when treated with antidepressants.

4.   Tricyclic antidepressants may foster "kindling" in bipolar patients, resulting in more rapid cycling.

5.   Do not rule out mania if elation and euphoria are not present. Sometimes the prominent affects are irritability and hostility. Manics, not schizophrenics, are the most hostile patients encountered by psychiatrists.

TRIVIA:

1.   Physicians of ancient Rome discovered that the waters of certain natural spas in northern Italy would sooth agitated or euphoric patients. Over 2000 years later these waters were found to be rich in lithium salts.

2.   "Mania" comes from the Greek root meaning "to be mad."

REFERENCES

1.   Akiskal HS: Affective disorders. In Merck Manual of Diagnosis and Therapy, 14th ed., Philadelphia, Merck Sharp and Dohme Research Laboratories, 1982.
2.   American Psychiatric Association Task Force on Nomenclature and Statistics: Diagnostic and Statistical Manual of Mental Disorders, 3rd ed. (DSM-III). Amer Psychiatric Association, Washington, DC, 1980.
3.   Clayton PJ: The epidemiology of bipolar affective disorder. Comp Psychiat 22:31-43, 1981.
4.   Dunner DL, et al: Classification of bipolar affective disorder subtypes. Comp Psychiat 23:186-189, 1982.
5.   Grinspoon L: Psychiatry Update, Vol II, Washington, DC, American Psychiatric Press, 1983.

CASE 15: Mrs. J, a 37-year-old, white, married, housewife and mother of three, nervously presents to your office after referral by her gynecologist. His thorough work-up had disclosed no medical cause for her complaint of fatigue. She notes to you that she "just doesn't enjoy anything anymore."

The onset of the problem is vague but appears to have been about six years ago. About that time the family was having some financial stress and she and her husband were having marriage problems. "But that all ended years ago. I don't understand it. Now I have everything, but I just don't enjoy it." Occasionally she will feel good for a few days but that is unpredictable and never lasts. Her past hobbies of oil painting and needlework have been untouched for over five years: "I'm not interested in it anymore. I just don't care. I'm always tired. Even when something good happens, I still feel dumpy."

She is somber and tearful. Her speech is mildly underproductive, lacks inflection, and is interrupted twice by quiet crying. No psychotic features or significant psychomotor retardation are present and she denies insomnia, anorexia, difficulty concentrating, suicide thoughts, obsessions, or drug/alcohol abuse.

HISTORICAL CLUES:

Her husband relates that she functions well as a mother and housewife, has several friends, and rarely misses the weekly meeting of her bridge club. But, in their 20 years of marriage she has "always been weak, never had much self-confidence, and depends a lot on me and her parents."

QUESTIONS:

1. What is the diagnosis?

2. Of what benefit was the information obtained from her husband?

3. What would you suspect in Mrs. J's family history?

4. What treatment would you prescribe?

ANSWERS:

1.   Dysthymic Disorder (DSM-III, 300.40). Prior to DSM-III
      this disorder was known as "depressive neurosis." The
      problem is one of chronic depression which is less
      severe than a "major depression." Such patients
      commonly complain of loss of interest, little pleasure,
      and feeling low or blue. The problem is characteris-
      tically chronic (DSM-III requires a duration of at
      least two years), however, periods of normal mood
      lasting for a few days or weeks may occur.

2.   Mr. J's information adds a collateral source which
      confirms and solidifies the suspected diagnosis. Both
      her history and presentation are consistent with dys-
      thymic disorder. He clarifies that her daily house-
      hold and social functioning are only mildly impaired.
      This is consistent with the diagnosis, although
      impairment of a more moderate or even severe nature
      can occur. In addition, he describes her personality
      in terms that suggest dependency - a common premorbid
      personality in those with this disorder.

3.   A diagnosis of dysthymic disorder suggests nothing in
      particular about the family history. No style of
      parenting or family conditions have consistently or
      conclusively been linked with this disorder. In
      addition, no convincing evidence of genetic factors
      has been found.

4.   Antidepressant medication may prove helpful, yet its
      use in this group has proven much less effective than
      in the group of major depressions. Some contend that
      depressive disorders occur along a spectrum with the
      dysthymic depressions being the less severe and major
      depressions the more severe expressions of the same
      disorder. This would account for the observation that
      some dysthymics respond to antidepressant medication
      (but raises questions about the lack of genetic
      findings).
            A trial of medication is warranted but may not be
      sufficient. The fact that such depressions commonly
      begin in young adulthood suggests some role for psycho-
      dynamic conflict, faulty personality, and/or difficulty
      adapting to adult roles. Psychotherapy should be
      prescribed. This allows the best opportunity to
      address her chronic dependency, low self-confidence,
      and low self-esteem, and may clarify the marriage and
      childhood contributions to her condition.

PEARLS:

1. Most patients with dysthymic disorder never require hospitalization though some are seen in emergency rooms and/or are hospitalized following suicide attempts or in response to increased somatic complaints.

2. Most people with depression receive no treatment. Those who do usually receive it from their primary care physicians. Only a small percentage of the total are seen by psychiatrists.

3. Dysthymic disorder occurs in children and adolescents, though its manifestations in these age groups are more likely to involve negativity, withdrawal, poor school performance, and acting-out.

4. Insidious onset and chronic course are characteristic.

5. This is a common condition which occurs more frequently in women than men (2-3:1).

6. Those with chronic physical disorders, chronic life stress, and/or chronic substance abuse are at particular risk.

PITFALLS:

1. A "gray zone" separates dysthymic disorder from normal mood fluctuations. Generally, normal mood fluctuations are not as severe or frequent and result in no impairment of social or occupational functioning.

2. Patients with dysthymic disorder may not present with complaints of depression. Some may even deny being depressed. "Masked depressions" are those in which the affective disturbance may not be obvious, but the patient presents with weight loss, insomnia, chronic pain, or other somatic complaints.

3. The most difficult differential diagnosis involves separating dysthymic disorder from the personality disorders. Dysthymic disorder can occur in conjunction with any personality disorder; however, it is often confused with histrionic, borderline, dependent, and narcissistic personality disorders.

TRIVIA:

Hippocrates attributed depression to an abnormal flux of black bile or "melana" - thus, the term "melancholia."

REFERENCES

1.   American Psychiatric Association Task Force on Nomenclature and Statistics: Diagnostic and Statistical Manual of Mental Disorders, 3rd ed. (DSM-III). Amer Psychiatric Association, Washington, DC, 1980.
2.   Finlay-Jones R, Brown GW: Types of stressful life events and the onset of anxiety and depressive disorders. Psychological Med 11:803-815, 1981.
3.   Hirschfeld RMA, Klerman GL: Personality attributes in affective disorders. Amer J Psychiat 136:67, 1979.
4.   Klerman GL, Endicott J, Hirschfeld RMA: Neurotic depression. Amer J Psychiat 136:57, 1979.
5.   Weissman MM, Plusoff BA, Dimascio A, et al: The efficacy of drugs and psychotherapy in the treatment of acute depressive episodes. Amer J Psychiat 136:555-558, 1979.
6.   Young JE, Beck AT: Cognitive therapy: Clinical applications. In Short-Term Psychotherapies for Depression, ed. by Rush AJ. New York, Guilford Press, 1982.

<u>CASE 16</u>: "My wife is frigid, a real icebox. I've tried every trick I know (and, believe you me Doc, I know a lot) and nothing gets her excited. She never was all that great but at least she used to put on a good show about liking sex. Now, she just avoids me and, when I insist, its like she was some place else.

"Ya, we get along OK otherwise, although this sex thing has made it kind of tough. I like to keep active, you know what I mean? We've been married 3 years and its been real bad for about the past 9 months. We argue about it and all she says is 'I'm sorry, dear, but I just can't help it. I don't know what's wrong.'

"What does she do? Doc, she don't do nothing, that's what I'm trying to tell you. She don't get hot and eager like my other women. No noises. Nothing. But, most of the time, she don't even want to start. No, she don't get nervous or anything. It's like she just don't care. Me? No way, Doc! I'm pretty good - like I could get testimonials if I wanted.

"No, she's not been sick or anything. Drugs? You got to be kidding. I don't think this woman likes to have fun. She don't even drink. Actually, she just sits around the house and mopes most of the time - and talks to her mother on the phone. Ya, that's what she does best - mopes.

"I swear, if I hear `I'm sorry, dear' one more time out of her, I'm going to be sick."

CLINICAL CLUE:

> The 37-year-old husband produced this diatribe while his 25-year-old wife sat in the room, eyes averted, staring at the floor. He would answer all questions directed to her. She wouldn't talk. He couldn't be kept quiet.

QUESTIONS:

1. Identify the problem here.

2. Who "deserves" a diagnosis?

3. What "psychosexual dysfunction" is present?

4. What has caused her condition?

5. What is the treatment for this condition?

ANSWERS:

1.   Although the impulse is to chuck the husband from your
     office and comfort the wife for having to live with
     him, there is an expressed problem that has caused
     them both to come for help and that needs to be ad-
     dressed: the husband, eager for a sexual relation with
     his wife, finds her reticent.
          Although you don't know her perspective, at least
     she was willing to come to the appointment with him
     and thus presumably shares his concerns to some degree.

2.   Diagnostic fashion dictates that in such a case we
     attempt to identify a disorder of psychosexual func-
     tioning. Although that probably can be done, these
     situations are often clinically complex. Even if we
     define a "disorder" on the wife's part, we should be
     careful not to "blame" her for the problem. Rather,
     it might be more helpful to define the problem in
     terms of the interpersonal relationship between hus-
     band and wife, since there appears to be a breakdown
     at that level.
          The temptation is strong to try to find a person-
     ality disorder diagnosis for the husband. Certainly
     distinct psychopathology should be looked for, yet his
     "outrageous" presentation may be merely a reaction to
     a personal life which he feels is out of control.

3.   We don't have enough information to be specific, but
     the most likely diagnosis is <u>inhibited sexual desire</u>
     on the part of the wife. He claimed that she was
     "frigid" (ie, was unable to become sexually excited
     physiologically - "inhibited sexual excitement" by
     DSM-III) but, in fact, the primary disorder may be one
     step earlier in the sexual response cycle. She may
     not become sexually aroused because she has little
     sexual desire.
          We need to ask her if that is the case. Further-
     more we need to determine if such a lack of interest
     applies only to her husband or is generalized to all
     sexual activity. Does she retain a normal spectrum of
     sexual fantasies? (In fact, when interviewed without
     her husband present, she admitted that she has had
     little sexual interest of any kind for at least the
     past year.)

4.   Possible causes for generalized impairment of sexual
     desire are numerous and include:
               <u>Biological causes</u> - chronic illness (eg, diabetes,
                    metabolic disorders, renal failure, etc),
                    drug abuse (particularly narcotics), alcohol-

ism (although moderate alcohol use often stimulates desire while impairing physiological responses), pregnancy and lactation.

Interpersonal causes - serious conflicts in the relationship between the two individuals: resentment, anger, etc.

Intrapersonal causes - "neurotic" conflicts about sexuality, certain severe personality disorders characterized by impaired intimacy (eg, schizoid, paranoid, narcissistic), fear of pregnancy or sexual disease, unusual sexual object choice (eg, wife who has a primary homosexual orientation), performance anxiety (more common among males, yet women may stifle desire when uncertain about their ability to perform satisfactorily).

Cultural causes - certain groups discourage sexual activity by labeling it "dirty" or otherwise unacceptable.

Psychiatric causes - many serious psychiatric illnesses can impair desire but most common are depression, anxiety, and reactions to stress.

We have insufficient information to explain the impaired desire in this case, yet we can make an educated guess as to its etiology. The marital relationship is rocky and the wife may harbor resentment and anger over the insensitivity and domineering ways of her husband. Perhaps of equal importance, however, is the fact that she appears significantly depressed. Depression is probably the most common psychiatric cause of generalized loss of sexual interest and, since her loss seems to be global, may well play a central role here. (In fact, she brightened up considerably after a trial of antidepressants and her general interest in sex returned. However, it benefited her husband little since, with her new found energy, she divorced him.)

5. Treatment depends upon the cause. Since the causes for impairment of sexual desire are legion, a variety of therapies may be useful: couple therapy, individual psychotherapy, medications, appropriate medical interventions, and specific behavioral methods.

PEARLS:

1. Impaired sexual desire is probably the most common type of sexual dysfunction (40% of patients in some sex clinics).

2.   Interpersonal anger is the most common cause of impaired sexual desire.

3.   It is possible, although not typical, for someone to have impaired desire yet display the full spectrum of physiological responses to genital stimulation.

4.   In certain cases, impairment of sexual desire can be very treatment resistant. The prognosis is most favorable if the patient has had high levels of desire in the past and if the loss is not generalized.

5.   Sexual desire is directly related to levels of plasma testosterone in males and levels of testosterone and androstendione in females. Estrogen decreases sexual desire in men.

PITFALLS:

It is a mistake to think that impairment of desire, or most other sexual dysfunctions, can be reversed by a simple regimen of "sex therapy exercises." Many of these conditions have complex roots and require a many-pronged therapeutic approach.

TRIVIA:

Anticipating modern science, Shakespeare said that drink "provokes the desire, but it takes away the performance."

REFERENCES

1. Bancroft J: Human Sexuality and Its Problems. London, Churchill Livingstone, 1983.
2. Bancroft J, Sanders D, et al: Mood, sexuality, hormones and the menstrual cycle III. Sexuality and the role of androgens. Psychosom Med 45:509, 1983.
3. Cole M: Sex therapy - A critical appraisal. Brit J Psychiat 147:337-351, 1985.
4. Davidson JM, Chen JJ, et al: Hormonal changes and sexual function in aging men. J Clin Endocrinol Metab 57:71, 1983.
5. Kaplan HS: Disorders of Sexual Desire. Washington, DC, American Psychiatric Press, 1985.
6. Kwan M, Greenleaf WJ, et al: The nature of androgen action on male sexuality: A combined laboratory, self-report study on hypogonadal men. J Clin Endocrinol Metab 57:557, 1983.
7. Persky H, Dreisbach L, et al: The relation of plasma androgen levels to sexual behaviors and attitudes of women. Psychosom Med 44:305-318, 1982.

CASE 17: A 67-year-old hardware supply store owner was brought for evaluation by his wife because his behavior had become increasingly peculiar over the past year.

At first he was just more irritable than normal: his usually placid disposition was replaced by constant criticism, mutterings, and ruminations. Old friends found him hard to get along with. Then he began to get his billings at work confused with the home finances. He would misplace things, forget appointments, and recently had even had trouble making change for customers. He became angry when he, or someone else, noticed these errors. In fact, he lost his temper over even the most minor events. He seemed to be changing in other ways as well. Always immaculate and compulsive, he became sloppy and careless. He often appeared lost in thought and he had become noticeably more forgetful.

More upsetting to the family, however, have been the suspicions he had developed over the past four months. He had gradually become convinced that his wife, children, and neighbors were responsible for his recent troubles. To him, his mislaid garden tools had been stolen by formerly close neighbors. His office books hadn't balanced because his son had been taking money from the till. Worst of all, his wife of 45 years was "cheating on him."

In fact, the immediate episode leading to evaluation was a battle between the patient and his wife in which he demanded that she admit her infidelities. Meanwhile, in frustration, she trotted her husband's recent ineptitudes and peculiarities before him. The family had finally "had enough" and, in an effort to protect the mother from this "crazy man," brought him to the psychiatrist.

PSYCHOBIOLOGICAL CLUE:

The majority of central acetylcholine (cholinergic) neurons are of three types: output motor neurons from the motor cortex and the cranial nuclei; caudate and putamen neurons involved with the extrapyramidal system; and basal forebrain neurons (from the nucleus basalis of Meynert) which innervate the cerebral cortex and the hippocampus. Both the cortex and hippocampus play central roles in human memory.

QUESTIONS:

1.   What is the obvious diagnosis?

2.   What should be considered in the differential diagnosis?

3.   How useful is psychological testing?

4.   How useful is laboratory and radiographic testing?

5.   What is the biological basis of this condition?

6.   Why was this patient paranoid?

ANSWERS:

1.   There is none. Too many individuals, including pro-
      fessionals, think peculiar behavior, failing memory,
      suspiciousness, altered personality, and other symp-
      toms are a natural part of growing older. They aren't!
      Likewise, some people assume that these changes in the
      elderly always indicate senile dementia. They don't!

2.   This patient's symptoms are consistent with many con-
      ditions and specific to none. Dementia, depression,
      atypical psychosis (eg, paraphrenia - a delusional
      condition presenting for the first time in late life)
      all need to be considered.
           In fact, he suffers from Primary Degenerative
      Dementia (DSM-III, 290.20) or Alzheimer's disease, the
      most common type of dementing illness. Whether it
      begins in the 40's, 50's, or 60's (formerly thought to
      be a distinct disease, presenile dementia) or in the
      70's, 80's, or 90's (formerly known as senile demen-
      tia), Alzheimer's disease is a relentlessly progres-
      sive biological illness characterized histologically
      by senile plaques, neurofibrillary tangles, and neuro-
      nal granulovacuolar degeneration in the cerebral
      cortex. The cause is unknown. Patients develop ob-
      vious symptoms of dementia (ie, a broad loss of intel-
      lectual functions) over a period of months or years.
      The diagnosis depends in part upon eliminating other
      causes of dementia. Depression, delirium, and other
      specific psychiatric illnesses should also be elim-
      inated as the primary cause of the symptoms. Thus,
      Alzheimer's disease is a diagnosis of exclusion. Be
      aware, however, that symptoms may be subtle and/or
      misleading at first (as in this case) and thus must
      always be thought of in the psychiatrically impaired
      elderly. On the other hand, don't over-diagnose.

3.   Essential. Some form of formal mental status testing
      should be performed whenever the diagnosis of a demen-
      tia is being considered. Comprehensive testing such
      as the Halstead and Reitan Batteries are too time
      consuming to be used routinely, but numerous brief
      examinations of mental status are available. It is
      essential, however, that each of the key areas of pos-
      sible dysfunction be tested: memory, cognition, affect,
      language, and behavior. On the other hand, subtleties
      such as altered judgment or social perception may be
      missed if psychological testing is exclusively relied
      upon to make the diagnosis of dementia. There is no
      substitute for a comprehensive psychiatric exam.

4. Essential. Both types of tests are crucial for ruling in or out other causes of dementia or dementia-like conditions. A CT scan is particularly useful.

5. Unknown. However, there is suggestive evidence that a primary degeneration of the cholinergic neurons in the Nucleus Basalis of Meynert may play a role. These neurons innervate the cerebral cortex and hippocampus. Their degeneration could account for the senile plaques and reduced choline acetyltransferase activity found in cortical biopsies of Alzheimer patients.

6. Delusions, hallucinations, and other psychiatric symptoms not usually associated with dementia occur from time to time and can be quite misleading. Their sole purpose seems to be to keep psychiatrists on their toes.

PEARLS:

1. The diagnosis of Alzheimer's disease can be made unequivocably only by brain biopsy or at autopsy.

2. Alzheimer's disease is the fourth leading cause of death in people over 65.

3. The earlier the onset, the more rapid the course is likely to be. The average life expectancy after onset is eight years, but death can follow as quickly as 1-2 years.

4. Molecular immunochemical similarities reported recently between Alzheimer's disease and the much rarer Pick's disease lend weight to the growing suspicion that these two disorders may be variants of a common pathologic process.

5. Down's syndrome patients over the age of 30 have an increased risk of developing the histopathological changes characteristic of Alzheimer's disease.

PITFALLS:

1. Don't predict how long your patient will live. Although Alzheimer's disease typically runs a steady downhill course, there are enough exceptions and cases with prolonged plateaus (for unknown reasons) to make prediction risky.

2. Social skills often are preserved in early Alzheimer patients. Don't miss the diagnosis by neglecting formal mental status testing in the patient who presents himself well socially.

3. Never accept significant late-life changes in memory, cognition, affect, or behavior as normal or as "just senility."

REFERENCES

1. Barclay LL, Zemcov A, Blass JP, McDowell FH: Factors associated with duration of survival in Alzheimer's disease. Biol Psychiatry 20:86-93, 1985.
2. Coyle JT, Price DL, DeLong MR: Alzheimer's disease: A disorder of cortical cholinergic innervation. Science 219:1184-1190, 1983.
3. Eslinger PJ, Damasio AR, Benton AL, Van Allen M: Neuropsychologic detection of abnormal mental decline in older persons. JAMA 253:670-674, 1985.
4. Katzman R: Alzheimer's disease. NEJM 314:964-973, 1986.
5. Price DL, Cork LC, et al: The functional organization of the basal forebrain cholinergic system in primates and the role of this system in Alzheimer's disease. In Olter DS, Gamzu E, Corkin S: Memory Dysfunction, New York, Annals New York Academy of Sciences, 1985.
6. Reisberg B: Alzheimer's Disease: The Standard Reference. New York, The Free Press, 1983.
7. Sims NR, Bowen DM, et al: Presynaptic cholinergic dysfunction in patients with dementia. J Neurochem 40:503-509, 1983.
8. Wolozen BL, Pruchnicki A, Dickson DW, Davis P: A neuronal antigen in the brains of Alzheimer patients. Science 232:648-650, 1986.

CASE 18: A 34-year-old woman who carried a diagnosis of panic disorder and who had suffered sudden episodes of palpitations, dyspnea, dizziness, and apprehension for several years appeared in the emergency room in the midst of a severe bout of her illness. She described feeling panicky and "as if her heart were about to jump out of her chest."

The intern contacted the patient's physician, a psychiatrist, who advised hospitalization on the psychiatric ward. However, after a careful physical examination and a stat ECG, the intern elected to admit the patient directly to the CCU. He was later heard to mutter, "That's just what you would expect from a psychiatrist."

CLINICAL CLUE:

On auscultation, the intern heard a nonejection, mid-systolic click and a soft, apical, late systolic murmur. The ECG showed T wave inversions in leads II, III, and aVF along with S-T segment depression.

QUESTIONS:

1. What mechanism probably produced the "click?"

2. What mechanism probably produced the murmur?

3. What is another name for this "click-murmur syndrome?"

4. Should this woman have been rushed to the CCU?

5. Was this syndrome responsible for the patient's symptoms?

6. Should the intern be required to take an additional rotation through the psychiatry service?

ANSWERS:

1. The ballooning of loose mitral valve leaflets into the left atrium during systole is "brought up short" by the sudden tensing of the chordae tendinae and surrounding anatomical structures, producing a "click."

2. The distended and compromised mitral valve permits flow of blood into the left atrium, producing a murmur of mitral regurgitation.

3. Mitral Valve Prolapse (MVP).

4. Probably not. Although "clicks and murmurs," when heard in the context of a panicky patient, can be alarming, mitral valve prolapse is usually asymptomatic and benign.

5. Probably not. The relationship between MVP and panic symptoms is not well understood. There seems to be an association since approximately 20% of patients with Panic Disorder (DSM-III 300.01) have MVP and more than 10% of MVP patients have panic disorder. However, the strength of this association has been weakened by the growing evidence that MVP is very common in the general population (5% of the population and perhaps as much as 17% in certain groups such as young females).

   Pointing towards an association is the fact that, although most patients with MVP are asymptomatic, the symptoms that do occasionally occur can mimic those of panic disorder: palpitations, dyspnea, weakness, chest pain, fatigue, syncope, dizziness, anxiety and a sense of panic. Moreover, both disorders are familial and occur about twice as often in women.

   On the other hand, no mechanism relating the two conditions has been identified. Nor does successful treatment of either condition (eg, panic disorder treated with imipramine or MVP treated with propranolol) usually influence the other disorder.

   So, we are left with two conditions which may occur together with a frequency greater than chance and which share certain epidemiologic features, but which don't seem to have a major influence on one another. They should be treated independently and their combined occurrence in one person should currently be viewed just as an interesting finding.

6. No. Rather, he should repeat cardiology for "over-reading" a midsystolic click.

PEARLS:

1.   Approximately 10% of patients in cardiology clinics
     present with symptoms that are primarily psychiatric
     in nature - commonly symptoms of anxiety and panic.

2.   Easy fatigability and exercise intolerance occurs with
     both MVP and panic disorder, but probably through
     different mechanisms.

3.   There is a growing suspicion that the panic-like sym-
     toms found in some MVP patients may be related to an
     increased alpha-adrenergic tone often found in these
     patients; the increased tone apparently caused by some,
     as yet unidentified, central (diencephalic) pathology.

4.   The diagnosis of MVP usually can be confirmed by echo-
     cardiography - only rarely is cardiac catheterization
     required, and then only in the most symptomatic
     patients.

PITFALLS:

     Just as it is a mistake to overlook medical syndromes
     when treating a psychiatric illness, so it is an error
     to neglect a psychiatric illness when treating a
     medical condition.

REFERENCES

1.   Crowe RR: Mitral valve prolapse and panic disorder. In
     Anxiety Disorders, ed. by Curtis GC, Thyer BA, Rainey
     JM, The Psychiatric Clinics of North America, Phila-
     delphia, WB Saunders, 1985.
2.   Evans DL, Kalina K: Effect of phenelzine on the pro-
     lapsed mitral valve in a patient with agoraphobia with
     panic attacks. J Clin Psychopharmacol 3:36-38, 1983.
3.   Gonzalez ER: The "nonneurotic" approach to mitral
     valve prolapse (Medical News). JAMA 246:2113-20, 1981.
4.   Hartmen N, Kramer R, Brown WT, Devereux RB: Panic dis-
     order in patients with mitral valve prolapse. Am J
     Psychiatry 139:669-670, 1982.
5.   Liberthson R, Sheehan DV, et al: The prevalence of
     mitral valve prolapse in patients with panic disorders.
     Am J Psychiat 143:511-515, 1986.
6.   Nishimura RA, McGoon MD, et al: Echocardiographically
     documented mitral-valve prolapse. NEJM 313:1305-1309,
     1985.
7.   Szmuilowicz J, Flannery JG: Mitral valve prolapse syn-
     drome and psychological disturbance. Psychosomatics
     21:419-421, 1980.

CASE 19: The Chairman of the Department of Surgery asks you to evaluate a 3rd year resident who is about to be dismissed from the program. The chairman is perplexed as to why this obviously capable young physician can't "get his act together" but, when asked what the trouble seems to be, he says "Wait until you meet him." Apparently, although bright and competent, the resident has managed to so alienate the surgery faculty, his peers, the hospital staff, and many of his patients that the clear departmental consensus is that he has no future in surgery.

The resident agrees readily to the interview. He arrives at your office promptly. He is pleasant, handsome, well-spoken, and immaculately dressed. He indicates that he has half expected such an interview for a long time because the surgery department has never really known what to make of him and sooner or later would need to call in an expert.

Asked to elaborate, he describes himself as being "at least two cuts above the other residents" and a match for any of the junior faculty. The senior faculty has never had to deal with anyone of his ability before in a training capacity and thus have viewed his "natural collegial relationship" with them as arrogance. He then recites a string of examples of his technical superiority and intellectual prescience to document his case.

When asked to address the specific complaints of the Surgery Residency Review Committee that he was brusque and unhelpful with students, far too willing to allow others to assume his clinical responsibilities when on call, and routinely caustic or belittling when challenged on his judgment or knowledge, he dismisses their objections with a wave of his hand. He then replies that he can't be bothered with issues peripheral to his own development: time is short and, although his rise has been meteoric to this point, he has much to do before his abilities are widely recognized. To the complaint that his rapport with patients is unusually poor, he notes that patients tire him but then they don't appreciate that no one in the department is more capable of handling truly difficult technical problems.

His past personal and family history is negative for psychiatric illness although he points out, with apparent satisfaction, that he has had "trouble" like this throughout his academic career.

A complete mental status examination is unremarkable. A detailed search for evidence of hallucinations, delusions, or formal thought disorder is unproductive.

CLINICAL CLUE:

By the end of the interview he has become testy.   Upon leaving, he says "I don't know what a shrink can add to what I've already told the chairman."

QUESTIONS:

1.   Is this man psychotic?

2.   Did he have insight into his "condition?"

3.   How do you reconcile his nice appearance and pleasant attitude toward you with the reports that he is caustic and belittling with others?

4.   What is the diagnosis?

5.   Is treatment indicated in this case?

ANSWERS:

1.   No. The term "psychotic" implies a <u>gross</u> impairment
      of reality testing - ie, misperception to a delusional
      degree. This man clearly thinks overly well of him-
      self but his justification, although distorted, is
      within reason and thus does not represent psychosis.
      Therefore we cannot make the diagnosis of a psychia-
      tric condition, such as schizophrenia, that requires
      psychosis to be part of the clinical picture.
          After considerable searching, no delusions,
      hallucinations, or formal thought disorder were found,
      further substantiating the absence of psychosis.

2.   He had very little real insight. ("Insight" is rarely
      <u>totally</u> absent or totally present.) Although he was
      aware that others considered him arrogant, he was not
      offended by this but, rather, considered such apparent
      "jealousy" on their parts to be an understandable
      fallout from his natural superiority. (In fact, for
      the three years of his residency this man was the butt
      of innumerable jokes among the medical students - as
      he shouldered his way throughout the hospital, his
      domineering ways were described as "the perfect
      personality for a surgeon," much to the chagrin of his
      fellow surgical residents.

3.   You were new to him, had a reputation as an "expert,"
      and gave him your full attention. By the time the
      interview was over, he was used to you and had "de-
      valued" you in comparison to himself as just a
      "shrink."
          The reports of people who have had prolonged
      contact with him are probably better measures of the
      quality of his interpersonal relationships.

4.   Narcissistic personality disorder (DSM-III, 301.81).
      These patients are intrusively grandiose, haughty,
      egocentric, exhibitionistic, exploitative of others,
      and condescending. (This patient displayed all of
      these characteristics.) Moreover, they are indiffer-
      ent to the feelings of others but frequently respond
      with anger or rage ("narcissistic rage") when they are
      treated in a cavalier fashion themselves.
          Although these patients are clinically distinct,
      the etiology of their disorder is unknown. Psycho-
      analytic metapsychological theories abound, however,
      which explain the condition in terms of early child-
      hood relationships. The validity of these explanations
      remains to be proven.

5.   This patient is neither asking for treatment nor likely to accept it. Instead, he came "readily" for an evaluation because he was seeking and expecting validation of his assumed superiority from an expert. Treatment of these individuals, when successful, is typically lengthy and requires at least a modicum of willing participation from the patient.

PEARLS:

1.   Content with themselves and condescending towards others, people with narcissistic personality disorder do not usually seek treat voluntarily.

2.   The increase in the incidence of narcissistic personality disorder has been attributed by some to the rise of the "me generation" (eg, see Lasch). It is unlikely, however, that a short-term change in cultural values has altered the incidence of a profound pathological condition of personality organization.

3.   These patients typically have a "corruptible conscience": they automatically shift their values to match their needs and desires. Thus, they can mimic the patient with an antisocial personality disorder.

4.   Some therapists argue that underneath the arrogant, self-assured, grandiose exterior of the narcissist lies a deeper personality that is envious, uncertain, and fearful and which is fundamentally responsible for the intrusive ways of these patients. Although this conceptualization remains theoretical, it is supported by the clinical observation that these individuals frequently become depressed and are often plagued by feelings of insecurity and inadequacy.

PITFALLS:

This condition is recognized more frequently today than a decade ago. (Although the diagnosis is new in DSM-III, psychiatrists have been aware of the clinical picture for many years.) This increase is probably due to diagnostic "fashion" rather than to a real rise in incidence.

REFERENCES

1. Akhtar L, Thomson JA: Overview: Narcissistic personality disorder. Am J Psychiat 139:12-20, 1982.
2. Ansbacher HL: The significance of Alfred Adler for the concept of narcissism. Am J Psychiat 142:203-206.
3. Goldstein WN: DSM-III and the narcissistic personality. Am J Psychotherapy 39:4-16, 1985.
4. Lasch C: The Culture of Narcissism. New York, WW Norton & Co., 1979.
5. Millon T: Disorders of Personality. New York, John Wiley & Sons, 1981.
6. Svrakic DM: Emotional features of narcissistic personality disorder. Am J Psychiat 142:720-7724, 1985.

CASE 20: A 28-year-old truck driver presents to the office of a psychiatrist. The patient is emotionally cold and aloof, stating only that he is there because "his wife is upset." It becomes clear that he has come on his wife's insistence and he has little personal interest in the appointment. He refuses the doctor's request to contact his wife, but says he will come again "in a few weeks." On the second visit he arrives 15 minutes late, talks somewhat more freely, but still displays anger and resentment about being forced to come. He admits to marriage problems and numerous depressive symptoms. Imipramine (cautiously built to 200 mg PO QHS) is prescribed. He reluctantly agrees to weekly psychotherapy and "maybe" marriage therapy in the future. After a month, his symptoms have shown no improvement despite an increase of the imipramine to 300 mg a day.

His medication is changed to amitriptyline due to his nonresponse and his repeated complaint of insomnia. After one month of 300 mg/day, he reports no benefit, no side effects, and complains of getting no help from the doctor. He still refuses the doctor any contact with his wife. Over the next few months similar failures result from seemingly adequate trials on maprotiline and doxepin. When it is suggested that he try an MAO inhibitor, the patient storms out of the office, never to return.

LABORATORY CLUE:

Plasma levels of the doxepin/nordoxepin were taken on three occasions. Date, dosage, and plasma levels were as follows: 6/14, 200 mg/day, 40 ng/ml; 6/29, 300 mg/day, 20 ng/ml; 7/10, 400 mg/day, 30 ng/ml (therapeutic range = 100-200 ng/ml).

QUESTIONS:

1. What likely accounts for this lack of response to the medication?

2. How common is this problem?

3. What patient factors and characteristics are commonly associated with this problem?

4. What physician factors and characteristics tend to decrease this problem?

ANSWERS:

1.   All indications are that the patient is not complying
      with the prescribed treatment. The patient's hostile
      attitude, complaints about the doctor, nonresponse to
      medications, lack of side effects, and low plasma
      levels in spite of very high supposed dosage are all
      clues that the medication is not being taken as pre-
      scribed. The fact that higher doses produced lower
      plasma levels is also inconsistent. Other possibili-
      ties such as poor absorption, rapid metabolism, and
      misdiagnosis or wrong medication should be considered
      but all seem remote possibilities compared to the more
      common problem of noncompliance.

2.   It is estimated that 25-50% of medical patients and
      40-50% of psychiatric patients are noncompliant with
      prescribed treatment.

3.   Decreased compliance occurs most often in children;
      the elderly; prophylactic, rather than acute, treat-
      ment; diseases where decreased medication does not
      bring immediate unpleasant consequences; grandiose,
      paranoid, or hostile patients; patients who perceive
      little threat from their condition; confused or
      psychotic patients; those who deny or lack insight;
      and situations where treatment costs are high or where
      there is little family or social support.

4.   Compliance is greater when the physician believes in
      the importance and efficacy of the treatment he is
      prescribing. Correct diagnosis, adequate prescription
      of proper medication, and skillful supervision also
      contribute to compliance. The quality of the
      doctor/patient relationship also correlates positively
      with compliance. The "ideal" relationship fostering
      compliance is felt to be characterized by warmth,
      understanding, negotiation, some degree of patient
      control and responsibility, active patient participa-
      tion, and shared expectations. Communication has been
      shown to be optimal when it is relatively brief,
      avoids technical terms, presents the most important
      information first, and is accompanied by written
      information.

PEARLS:

1.   Noncompliance has a significant impact on health and
      treatment costs. It has been estimated that 20-25% of
      all hospitalizations result from noncompliance with
      prescribed outpatient regimens and that about 30% of

patients misuse their medication in ways that pose a danger to their health.

2. A patient's attitudes and beliefs about his illness are more potent determinants of compliance than are his actual education and technical level of understanding.

3. The "Health Belief Model" developed by Becker predicts patient compliance. It states that compliance with a particular therapy is associated with "the patient's perception of personal susceptability to an illness, the severity of the consequences of the condition, the potential benefits of therapy, and the financial, social and psychological costs of the therapy..." (Docherty, 1985).

4. Medication factors known to contribute to noncompliance are undesirable side effects, nonresponse, prescription of many drugs, many daily doses, long treatment duration, self-administration, oral route, and "childproof" safety packaging.

PITFALLS:

1. Studies repeatedly confirm that physicians' estimates of compliance/noncompliance are poor. A high level of awareness, collateral interviews, and objective measures such as blood levels and pill counts increase accuracy.

2. Not taking prescribed medication is only one type of noncompliance, though probably the most common type. Others are wrong time, wrong sequence, and wrong medication, as well as too much medication, undisclosed additional medications, or disregard of instructions in other ways.

3. Level of compliance is not a constant for a given patient. It varies with factors such as time, physician, relationship, illness, and treatment.

4. Compliance has not been shown to relate predictably to sex, race, education, social class, occupation, or marital status.

5. It is estimated that 35-50% of patients are dissatisfied with the communication with their physician and that they frequently forget or never understand information that has been presented.

TRIVIA:

Hippocrates warned physicians to "keep aware of the fact that patients often lie when they state that they have taken certain medicines."

REFERENCES

1. Asburn L: Patient compliance with medication regimens, in Biobehavioral Medicine, ed. by Ledcomb SJ, NSW, Cumberland College of Health Sciences, 1981.
2. Becker MH: Understanding patients compliance; The contributions of attitude and other psychosocial factors. In New Directions in Patient Compliance, ed. by Cohen SJ, Lexington MA, Heath & Co., 1979.
3. Docherty, JP, Fiestes SJ: The therapeutic alliance and compliance in psychopharmacology. In Psychiatry Update, Annual Review Volume IV. ed. by Hales E, Frances AJ. American Psychiatric Press, Washington, DC, 1985.
4. Evans L, Spelman M: The problem of noncompliance in drug therapy. Drugs 25:63-76, 1983.
5. Ley P: Satisfaction, compliance and communications. Br J Clin Psychol 21:241-234, 1982.

FAMILY FEUD

<u>CASE 21</u>: An 18-year-old, black, single female presented to the intake worker at the local community mental health center. She had recently been graduated from high school and expressed confusion about what to do with her life. "I'd like to go to college but my boyfriend is really pressuring me to get married. He works at the cement plant and wants me to take a job there answering the phone. He doesn't think college is important and neither do my parents."

She mentioned symptoms of increased irritability, mild initial insomnia, occasional crying spells, lethargy, mild withdrawal from friends, and impulses to run away. In recent weeks her father has become angry at her. In exasperation he yelled at her, "Stop thinking so much and just get married!" Her pastor suggested she get into some therapy at the mental health center. She did not take his suggestion very seriously, but after three weeks of increasing depression she decided to come to the mental health center and "check it out."

The intake worker felt that the problem was an Adjustment Disorder with Depressed Mood (DSM-III 309.00) and decided to make arrangements for her to begin psychotherapy.

QUESTIONS

1. In making this referral, what consideration should be given to the sex and race of the therapist?

2. What patient factors have correlated with successful psychotherapy outcome?

3. What therapist factors have correlated with successful psychotherapy outcome?

4. What professional discipline and amount of training and experience are correlated with successful outcome?

ANSWERS:

1.   Some researchers assert that progress in therapy is maximized when patient and therapist are of the same sex and that this matching may be particularly helpful for marital, sexual, identification, and adolescent problems. Though the practice is not widely accepted, research studies have generally favored pairing female patients with female therapists. In these studies, the benefit of this pairing was most marked in the therapy of women who were young, depressed, and single. Also, the majority of studies indicate that blacks feel better understood, form a more positive alliance, enter into more self-exploration, and respond better to therapy when working with a black therapist. It should be kept in mind that general trends shown in research studies do not predict what will happen with the individual patient. Also gender and race are only two of many variables in the psychotherapy setting and while important, they do not usually override such therapist factors as technical competance, empathy, and personality.

2.   Problem-solving attitude, capacity for experiencing, good premorbid adjustment, "likeability," motivation, activity in therapy, assumption of some responsibility for progress, and positive attitude toward the therapist have all correlated with psychotherapy success. Other factors linked to better outcome but not firmly demonstrated by research include the presence of a precipitating stress, the presence of strong emotion, the expectation of improvement, and higher intelligence. Psychologically healthier patients form more efficient working relationships and, as a group, do better in psychotherapy. Contrariwise, those who need therapy the most seem to improve the least with it.
      Factors often linked to poorer outcome are psychotic illness, preoccupation with physical symptoms, and marked hostility or defensiveness during early therapy sessions. Half of the studies show no association between age and outcome while half identify greater improvement in younger patients.
      After almost 100 years of research and practice, the question of who is most suitable for and most benefits from psychotherapy remains incompletely answered.

3.   Empathy and competant technical performance in the therapist have correlated with psychotherapy success in recent well-designed research studies. Other

therapist qualities which "sound logical" but which are not proven to be important include warmth (genuine concern), congruence (words matching feelings), flexibility, sensitivity, maturity, intelligence, imaginativeness, and self-confidence. Some (most notably the followers of Carl Rogers' client-centered therapy) support the idea that warmth, empathy, and genuineness are sufficient attributes independent of training or other qualifications. Most would accept the importance of these factors yet disagree that they provide sufficient conditions in the therapist.

Attempts to define and investigate therapist expertise have been largely unsuccessful. Indicators are that the relationship and personal factors brought to therapy by the patient are more closely correlated to outcome than those contributed by the therapist.

4.   None has been shown to be related to outcome.

PEARLS:

1.   Most providers of psychotherapy are men while most patients are women.

2.   Minorities and members of lower socioeconomic classes enter into therapy less frequently and remain in therapy for shorter periods.

3.   A person's past experiences and relationships with parents and other important people in their life is the most consistent determinant of their ability to form a working therapeutic alliance with a therapist.

4.   Patients who are liked by their therapist have better outcomes in psychotherapy. This finding may parallel the demonstration of better school performance in students who are liked by their teachers.

PITFALLS:

1.   Studies have shown correlation between psychological disturbance in the therapist and poor outcome in the patient.

2.   Racial biases and stereotypes have been demonstrated in about 75% of therapists.

TRIVIA:

The typical patient in psychotherapy during the time of Freud was educated, young, middle-class, neurotic, and female. The uneducated and people past about 45 years old were largely regarded as untreatable.

REFERENCES

1. Black C: Diagnostic and treatment issues for black patients. The Clin Psychologist 37:51-54, 1984.
2. Bloch S: What Is Psychotherapy?. New York, Oxford University Press, 1982.
3. Blumenthal SJ, et al: The influence of gender and race on the therapeutic alliance. In Psychiatric Update: Annual Review, Vol. IV, ed. by Hales RE, Frances AJ. American Psychiatric Association, Wash, DC, 1985.
4. Harrison JK: Race as a counselor-client variable in counseling and psychotherapy: A review of the research. The Counseling Psychologist 5:124-133, 1975.
5. Jones EE, Zoppel C: Input of client and therapist gender on psychotherapy process and outcome. J Consult Clin Psychol 50:259-272, 1982.
6. Morgan R, et al: Predicting the outcome of psychotherapy by the Penn Helping Alliance Rating Method. Arch Gen Psychiatry 39:397-402, 1982.

DRY SCHIZOPHRENIA

CASE 22: Mrs. J, a 77-year-old, white, widowed female was brought to the emergency room by her daughter. The daughter explained that Mom "seemed fine" during her last visit three days ago, but this morning she arrived to find her sitting unclothed on the floor, clinging and talking rapidly to a dirty towel. She would not allow any clothing to be placed on her. Any attempts were met by her tearing at the clothing and screaming, "Get them away, get them away!" With the help of a neighbor she was wrapped in a blanket and forced into the car for the trip to the hospital.

Past history did not seem helpful. Mrs. J had lived alone since her husband's death four years ago. She had no previous psychiatric problems and had always seemed to be happy and well adjusted. She had been in good health except for what seemed to be minor complaints such as morning stiffness in her right hip and occasional trouble sleeping.

On mental status she presented as grossly confused and unable to respond logically to any questions. She appeared agitated and emotionally labile, often picking at her hospital gown and screaming, "Get them away."

The emergency room intern diagnosed the patient as schizophrenic. He administered Thorazine 50 mg IM in an effort to settle her until the psychiatric resident arrived.

PHYSICAL EXAMINATION CLUES:

Temperature - 103.4°F. Pulse - 125/min and regular. BP - 145/60. Pupils - dilated and unreactive. Skin - warm and dry. Bowel sounds - absent.

QUESTIONS:

1. Was schizophrenia the correct diagnosis?

2. The past history was reported as "not helpful." Do you agree?

3. On careful physical examination, what other physical findings would you expect to be present?

4. What response would you expect from the dose of Thorazine (50 mg IM)?

5. What is the proper treatment?

ANSWERS:

1. No. In fact, there is very little in the history and presentation that suggests schizophrenia. The response by some physicians that "anything looking bizarre is schizophrenia" is both incorrect and potentially dangerous. This patient's history is of a rapid onset psychosis in a previously healthy elderly woman. The presentation is most consistant with delirium - confusion, agitation, and visual hallucinations. The physical examination reveals signs consistent with anticholinergic toxicity (warm, dry skin; dilated pupils; absent bowel sounds; hypotension; hyperpyrexia).

    Belladonna, scopolamine, atropine, and the antihistamines are commonly encountered in both prescription and over-the-counter preparations. In addition, many common prescription medications have anticholinergic potency (tricyclic antidepressants, antipsychotics, benztropine, dicyclomine, and many others). An overdose or unusual sensitivity may produce a medical picture called "anticholinergic delirium" or "central anticholinergic syndrome." This is characterized by disorientation, confusion, agitation, and impaired memory, with incoherence and a fluctuating level of sensorium. The physical signs of cholinergic blockade or sympathetic overactivity are invariably present as well.

    This problem is of special interest and concern in the elderly. Older individuals appear to be more vulnerable to the central effects of anticholinergics. Also, many self-medicate with a variety of agents which have some anticholinergic activity. Early symptoms of anticholinergic intoxication such as agitation or insomnia may be "treated" by taking more of the offending agent and thus compound the problem.

    Mrs. J's delirium was later found to be secondary to Sominex (scopolamine). Her arthritic pain had caused her trouble sleeping. She obtained the pills and when one didn't work the first night, she took two the next. It appeared that as she began to feel worse and became confused, she took increasing numbers of the pills. Two empty Sominex boxes were found in her home.

2. The past history is, in fact, quite helpful. Good premorbid adjustment and no previous psychiatric history essentially rules out schizophrenia. Schizophrenia does not erupt suddenly in the elderly. By DSM-III criteria, schizophrenia always begins before age 45. Also, her apparent good premorbid medical health tends

to rule against a variety of possible chronic medical conditions as the etiology of her delirium.

3. Dry mucus membranes, foul breath, flushed face, photophobia, and ataxia. Urinary retention and constipation are also likely to be present.

4. This was an extremely bad treatment choice, producing a situation of "everything to lose and nothing to win." Even if the diagnosis of schizophrenia was correct, this dose is excessive, considering the patient's age. Producing a state of severe hypotension is a very real and dangerous possible consequence. In addition, chlorpromazine is strongly anticholinergic. It would be expected to exacerbate and prolong her anticholinergic delirium. A risk is the creation a vicious cycle: misdiagnosis and mistreatment result in increased agitation and confusion, leading to higher doses of chlorpromazine.

5. Close supportive medical supervision and abstinence from the offending agent will usually reverse the condition in a few days. Physostigmine (1-4 mg IM or IV, every 30-60 minutes) may quickly reverse the symptoms and prove useful both in diagnosis and treatment. This approach is not without its own potential problems. Physostigmine (an anticholinesterase agent) has been known to cause heart block, excessive salivation with bronchoconstriction, and seizures.

PEARLS:

1. Anticholinergic agents are responsible for a large number of drug-induced psychiatric complications each year.

2. Anticholinergic agents are included in numerous over-the-counter preparations - cough syrups, decongestants, tranquilizers, and hypnotics.

3. Abuse of anticholinergic agents for their hallucinogenic effects is becoming more frequent.

4. When visual hallucinations are present, think first of an organic disorder.

5. Fatalities in anticholinergic overdoses are rare. Overdoses as high as 1000 mg of atropine have been survived.

6.   Pulse pressure is commonly widened in anticholinergic poisoning; ie, systolic pressure is raised and diastolic lowered.

7.   Belladonna alkaloids are contained in a variety of plants including jimson weed, devil's trumpet, angel's trumpet, and belladonna.

8.   In any patient who has had an acute onset of bizarre physical and mental symptoms, drug poisoning should be suspected.

PITFALLS:

In one study, 35% of patients over forty demonstrated some level of confusion while taking tricyclic antidepressants.

TRIVIA:

Centuries ago custom held that dark eyes were the most beautiful. A widely dilated pupil left only a narrow rim of colored iris, imparting the fashionable beauty of that era. Eye drops extracted from a common plant with reddish flowers and black berries became a necessity to every beautiful woman. The plant and its extract thus came to be called "belladonna" - beautiful lady.

REFERENCES

1.   Hall RCW, et al: Behavioral toxicity of non-psychiatric drugs. In Psychiatric Presentations of Medical Illness, ed. by Hall RCW. Spectrum Publications, NY, 1980.
2.   Hall RCW, et al: Angel's trumpet psychosis. Amer J Psychiatry 134:313-314, 1977.
3.   Jakobsen J, Hauksson P, Vestergaard P: Heart rate variation in patients treated with antidepressants: an index of anticholinergic effects? Psychopharmacology 84:544-48, 1984.
4.   Salzman C: A primer on geriatric psychopharmacology. Amer J Psychiatry 139:67-74, 1982.
5.   Weiner N: Atropine, scopolamine, and related antimuscarinic drugs. In Gilman AG, Goodman LS, et al (Eds.), The Pharmacological Basis of Therapeutics, New York, MacMillan Pub, 1985.

A STARTLING CASE

<u>CASE 23</u>: On a routine, bimonthly, nursing home visit a
university psychiatrist is introduced by the head nurse to
a new patient, Mr. L ("our newest Alzheimer's patient").
He is sitting in a chair and appears somewhat sedated. A
brief conversation with Mr. L shows him to be quite demented: although he can understand simple sentences and
respond to commands, he doesn't know the time, the day, or
his location, nor can he remember the psychiatrist's name
after one minute. As they are walking away, the nurse
comments: "That's the worse case of Alzheimer's disease I
have ever seen - he has gotten much worse during the four
weeks he has been here, and now he even has trouble
walking."

Realizing that he had taken too much for granted, the
psychiatrist returns to the patient and documents marked
upper and lower ataxia (poor finger-to-nose and heel-to-
shin performance and stumbling gait) and the presence of
occasional myoclonic jerks of his left arm and torso.
Then, when he stands behind the patient and suddenly claps
his hands, the patient jumps almost to a standing position.

The psychiatrist notes to the nurse that "that patient
doesn't have Alzheimer's disease," requests a thorough
laboratory evaluation including a CT scan and an EEG, and
then places a call to the nursing home's medical director.

Five weeks later, after transfer to the University
Hospital, the patient dies.

LABORATORY CLUE:

All laboratory evaluations and the CT scan were normal
but the EEG showed "diffuse, high-voltage sharp waves."

QUESTIONS:

1.   What was inconsistent with Alzheimer's disease?

2.   What did the psychiatrist say to the medical director?

3.   What was the point of the hand clapping that so star-
     tled the patient and so impressed the nurse with the
     psychiatrist's diagnostic acumen?

4.   What is the correct diagnosis?

5.   How can this diagnosis be confirmed?

ANSWERS:

1.   A patient with Alzheimer's disease rarely changes a
      great deal in only weeks - such a rapid course is
      strong evidence that some other process is present.
            Although a variety of neurological symptoms can
      accompany Alzheimer's disease, they are rarely as pre-
      dominant as they are in this patient.

2.   He suggested both that Mr. L had been diagnosed incor-
      rectly and that the condition from which he might be
      suffering was transmissible and possibly required low-
      level isolation precautions.

3.   A prominent characteristic of the condition he was
      considering is a strong startle response, particularly
      to loud noises.

4.   Creutzfeldt-Jakob disease.   One of the "myoclonic
      dementias," Creutzfeldt-Jakob disease usually presents
      in late middle age with dementia (loss of intelligence
      and memory) and emotional incontinence as well as with
      marked cerebellar ataxia and prominent myoclonic
      jerks.   If the dementia appears first, it may be
      mistaken for Alzheimer's disease until the motor fea-
      tures develop. However, it is a rapidly progressive
      dementing illness, so usually doesn't take long to
      declare itself (this patient went from uncomplicated
      dementia to death in about 2 months).
            Because it is rare (1:1,000,000), it is frequent-
      ly overlooked.

5.   The clinical picture of an aggressive dementia with
      profound ataxia and myoclonis is very suggestive, as
      is an EEG showing prominent, diffuse sharp waves.
      However, confirmation requires a tissue sample, pre-
      ferably from involved cerebral or cerebellar cortex.
            Gross pathology - characteristic but not diag-
      nostic - reveals diffuse deterioration across cortical
      areas. Micropathology, on the other hand, is unique
      in the extensive gliosis and the cytoplasmic vacuola-
      tion which gives the cortical tissue the appearance of
      a sponge and results in the general classification of
      this disease as a subacute spongiform encephalopathy.

PEARLS:

1.   Creutzfeldt-Jakob disease is felt to be a slow-virus
      encephalopathy related to scrapie in sheep and kuru in
      humans. It has been transmitted among chimpanzees and
      from humans to chimps. However, the presumptive

transmissible agent has not yet been found but is assumed to be a virus.

2.   This disorder can occur in "epidemics" and an "outbreak" (ie, several cases have been identified) has recently been noted among patients who have received "infected" human growth hormone extract.

3.   Although this disease is presumably infectious, strict isolation procedures are not required with patients.

PITFALLS:

1.   Creutzfeldt-Jakob disease occasionally can present first with bizarre ideas and behavior and be mistaken for an acute psychosis like schizophreniform disorder or mania.

2.   The disease has been transmitted by inadequately sterilized neurosurgical instruments.

REFERENCES

1.   Bendheim PE, Bockman JM, et al: Scrapie and Creutzfeldt-Jacob disease prion proteins share physical properties and antigenic determinants. Proc Natl Acad Sci USA 82:997-1001, 1985.

2.   Davanipour Z, Goodman L, et al: Possible modes of transmission of Creutzfeldt-Jakob disease. NEJM 311:1582-1583, 1984.

3.   Gibbs CJ, Joy A, et al: Clinical and pathological features and laboratory confirmation of Creutzfeldt-Jakob disease in a recipient of pituitary-derived human growth hormone. NEJM 313:734-738, 1985.

4.   Masters CL, Harris JO, et al: Creutzfeldt-Jakob disease: patterns of worldwide occurrence and the significance of familial and sporadic clustering. Ann Neurol 5:177-188, 1979.

5.   Masters CL, Gajdusek DC: The spectrum of Creutzfeldt-Jakob disease and the virus-induced spongiform encephalopathies. In Smith WT, Cavanagh JB (Eds.), Recent Advances in Neuropathology, No. 2. Edinburgh: Churchill-Livingstone, pp 139-163, 1982.

6.   Prusiner SB, Hadlow WJ: Slow Transmissible Diseases of the Nervous System. New York, Academic Press, 1979.

CASE 24: The patient is a 35-year-old married man who presented to the psychiatric outpatient department complaining of incapacitating anxiety.

He reported that about two years before, he had had a one-night homosexual affair. The following week, his wife developed a vaginal infection after having sexual intercourse with him. He then became very anxious, thinking that he had "given his wife a disease." In the days that followed he developed numbness of his right thigh, right-sided abdominal pain, and diarrhea and was admitted to a local hospital for evaluation. No organic etiology was found for any of his symptoms. The diagnosis of irritable bowel syndrome was made, he was started on Metamucil and a diet lacking milk products. Over the following months many of his symptoms disappeared although he continued to have stomach upset and mild diarrhea.

His anxiety became chronic and intrusive and was complicated by low-level feelings of depression. He couldn't sleep, "couldn't relax," was preoccupied with determining his "true sexual orientation," and was constantly worried lest his wife discover his sexual indiscretion. Various doctors prescribed various medications: antidepressants (imipramine, trazadone), minor tranquilizers (diazepam, alprazolam), and major tranquilizers (thorazine, haloperidol). The patient felt that these medications helped him sleep but otherwise were of little value.

Eight days before coming to the clinic, he caught his hand in some machinery at work. Although there was no serious injury, he became exceptionally anxious, broke down crying, couldn't be calmed, and had to leave. He spent the following eight days at home pacing, sobbing, and feeling too anxious to work or sleep.

In the clinic he appeared disheveled, agitated, and depressed but displayed no thought disorder, delusions, hallucinations, suicidal ideations, or memory impairment. He was cooperative but clearly uncomfortable and ill at ease. In the privacy of the consultation room, without his wife present, he blurted out the whole story ("I've never told this to anyone before, but I can't keep it to myself any longer"). He insisted that, in spite of his sobbing, he was troubled primarily by feelings of anxiety (without any specific focus) rather than by depression.

PSYCHOSOCIAL CLUE:

In the homosexual male, deviant urges and fantasies are almost always present in the late teenage years or the early twenties. The appearance of strong homosexual ideas "out of the blue" later in life is unusual.

QUESTIONS:

1. What are the most likely diagnoses for Axes I - III?

2. Why is depression not the primary diagnosis?

3. What medical conditions are most commonly or most clearly associated with anxiety symptoms?

4. Was the patient's isolated homosexual experience important to his problem?

5. What would be the most effective treatment for this patient?

ANSWERS:

1.   Axis I - Generalized anxiety disorder (DSM-III 300.02)
         Ego-dystonic homosexuality (DSM-III 302.00)

     Axis II - No diagnosis

     Axis III - Irritable bowel syndrome

     The patient qualified for generalized anxiety
disorder by virtue of a chronically anxious mood, agitation, autonomic hyperactivity (chronic diarrhea and upset stomach), and insufficient evidence to support a diagnosis of depression or schizophrenia.

2.   Anxiety patients frequently experience transient depressions, just as depressed patients are often anxious. Seen at the height of the depressed mood, patients with generalized anxiety disorder may be mistakenly felt to suffer from dysthymic disorder or major depression. However, over time it is the anxious affect which is continuous while the depression waxes and wanes. Thus the diagnosis (anxiety vs depression) hinges upon which group of symptoms is more prominent over time.
     On the other hand, the dividing line between the two disorders is often imprecise, both conditions may occur in the same individual, and as many as one third of seriously anxious patients develop a secondary depression. In fact, this patient noted a lifting of his feeling of depression and despair with a thorough trial of doxepin (his previous antidepressant trials had been brief and at low dosage) although he experienced little change in his anxiety.

3.   Although medical illnesses are often accompanied by anxiety, there are a few physical conditions which can produce anxiety as the primary symptom. However, they do so infrequently. Such "anxiety disorder mimics" include cardiovascular conditions like mitral valve prolapse and arrhythmias, hyperthyroidism, hypoglycemia, temporal lobe epilepsy, substance abuse, Cushing's disease, and mild delirious states.

4.   Yes! On further conversation (and after a degree of trust had developed between the patient and therapist), the patient confided that he had had several homosexual encounters over the years and that he was terrified that his homosexual urges might prove stronger than his love for his wife. This fear kept him in a state of near panic.

The patient's homosexual (actually, bisexual) orientation came as no surprise to the therapist, given the history of a "one time" homosexual encounter by the patient at age 35 (see the Psychosocial Clue).

5. As is the case in many other psychiatric conditions, the ideal treatment for any given patient with anxiety disorder is difficult to determine in advance.

Several medications may be useful. Benzodiazepines are the only sedative-hypnotics that should be used, and even they are not effective in every patient, often lose their effectiveness over time, and have some abuse potential. Antihistamines may be used to control anxiety symptoms in patients prone to abuse. The tricyclic antidepressants (particularly the more sedative ones such as amitriptyline and doxepin) and the MAO inhibitors may produce long-lasting improvement in a few patients (although those individuals likely to respond cannot be identified at this time). The beta-adrenergic blockers may help those patients in whom cardiovascular symptoms predominate.

Psychotherapy is frequently of greater value than medication. If an area of conflict (conscious or unconscious) appears to be central to anxiety production, approaching it directly through therapy is often useful. Relaxation techniques and meditation can help relieve symptoms. Support and reassurance is important in all anxious patients.

The patient above responded to a combination of approaches. Although his mood became brighter with doxepin, the majority of his symptoms began to abate only after he came to grips with his unwanted homosexual urges (ie, he had ego-dystonic homosexuality). Initially, however, the topic of his homosexuality was so anxiety producing that he needed to take a short acting benzodiazepine (alprazolam) before each session in order to have a productive conversation.

PEARLS:

1. Generalized anxiety disorder may not exist as a distinct entity. Rather, it may represent a diverse group of conditions of various etiologies having in common prominent anxiety.

2. Fewer than one third of patients with anxiety disorder fully recover.

3. Panic disorder runs in families and appears to have a genetic component, while generalized anxiety disorder does not (although this distinction has not been made to everyone's satisfaction).

4. Substance abuse (intoxication with stimulants; with-
    drawal from sedatives and alcohol) is the most common
    "medical" cause of anxiety. Look for it in the
    anxious patient who has abnormal liver function tests.

5. The tricky business of differentiating a primary
    anxiety disorder from a primary depression can be
    helped by sleep studies. Patients with anxiety dis-
    order show decreased stage I sleep and REM percentage
    while depressed patients typically show shortened REM
    latencies.

PITFALLS:

1. Because of the ubiquity of anxiety complaints among
    psychiatric patients, make the diagnosis of general-
    ized anxiety disorder cautiously - use the diagnosis
    "atypical anxiety disorder" when in doubt.

2. Be careful not to produce an iatrogenic addiction in
    the severely anxious patient who responds to (and
    wants) benzodiazepines. Over time, continuing anxiety
    may stem as much from low-level chronic withdrawal as
    from the initial anxiety disorder.

REFERENCES

1. Breier A, Charney DS, Heninger GR: The diagnostic
    validity of anxiety disorders and their relationship
    to depressive illness. Am J Psychiatry 142:787-797,
    1985.
2. Curtis GC, Thyer BA, Rainey JM: Anxiety disorders. The
    Psychiatric Clinics of North America, Vol 8, Number 1,
    Philadelphia, WB Saunders, March, 1985.
3. Fawcett J, Kravitz HM: Anxiety syndromes and their
    relationship to depressive illness. J Clin Psychiatry
    44 (8, Sec 2):8-11, August, 1983.
4. Insel TR, Ninan PT, et al: A benzodiazepine receptor-
    mediated model of anxiety. Arch Gen Psychiatry 41:741-
    750, 1984.
5. Shader RI, Greenblatt DJ: Some current treatment
    options for symptoms of anxiety. J Clin Psychiatry 44
    (11, Sec 2):21-29, November, 1983.
6. Togersen S: Genetic factors in anxiety disorders. Arch
    Gen Psychiatry 40:1085-1089, 1983.

CASE 25:   Mr. K's mother died of Huntington's disease when he was 23-years-old. He had several other afflicted relatives and knew that he had a 50-50 chance of developing the disease himself. Nevertheless, he married, had children, and hoped that the illness would miss him.

He was problem-free until age 43 when he developed a moderate depression that responded partially to antidepressant medication. A mild degree of depression and irritability persisted, however, over the following three years. Finally, the horror that had been at the back of his mind all these years came true: he began to develop choreiform movements. A diagnosis of Huntington's disease was made.

Over the following three years his movement disorder worsened, as did his depression. He became emotionally labile and was prone to bouts of acute depression as well as attacks of rage. His family life was in turmoil; not only because of his misbehavior but also because his children (3 boys and 1 girl; all teenagers) seemed to be reacting to their new awareness that now they each had a 50-50 chance of developing the disease they saw so terrifyingly displayed by their father.

In the midst of all this uproar, at age 49, Mr. K suddenly killed himself.

QUESTIONS:

1.   What do we know about the genetic transmission of Huntington's disease?

2.   Is it now possible to predict with certainty who will develop Huntington's disease?

3.   Should presymptomatic testing for Huntington's disease be made available to all HD family members?

4.   Is Huntington's disease a "cortical dementia?"

5.   What is the clinical significance of a subcortical dementia?

6.   Why did Mr. K become depressed before the onset of his neurological symptoms?

7.   What psychiatric symptoms are commonly associated with Huntington's disease?

ANSWERS:

1. Autosomal dominant transmission with complete pene-
    trance. Recent genetic work suggests that a single
    gene is involved, located on the short arm of chromo-
    some 4.   Children of affected parents have a 50%
    chance of developing the disease. First symptoms can
    appear anytime from childhood to the 70's but most
    frequently develop during a person's 30's or 40's.

2. No. A great variety of measures have been tried and
    have failed as presymptomatic indicators of HD. How-
    ever, modern genetics may change that. Although we
    are not yet able to identify the HD gene itself, we
    now recognize a particular genetic marker linked to
    that gene (a short DNA fragment located near the HD
    gene and known as the G8 probe). Unfortunately, such
    a linkage probe is not 100% accurate for the presence
    of the HD gene.

3. The ethical issues surrounding such testing are com-
    plex. The genetic linking test we now possess is too
    inaccurate to be used except in very special circum-
    stances - the effects of announcing results which turn
    out to be either false positives or false negatives
    are devastating.
        However, even if we are able to identify the HD
    gene with 100% accuracy, major ethical, legal, social,
    and psychological problems arise. Although it might
    always seem better for the individual "to know" than
    "not to know," how is the presymptomatic patient ex-
    pected to face life in a normal, vigorous, and healthy
    way knowing the years of hopeless incapacity that lie
    ahead?   If prenatal screening becomes available, as
    seems likely, how does one make social and legal deci-
    sions about a life that may be functional and healthy
    for decades before the illness becomes manifest?

4. Huntington patients eventually become demented. A
    distinction has been made recently between dementing
    conditions which affect primarily the cerebral cortex
    ("cortical dementias" such as Alzheimer's disease) and
    those that involve subcortical structures ("subcortical
    dementias" such as Huntington's disease, Parkinson's
    disease, and progressive supranuclear palsy). HD is
    characterized by cell loss (small, spiny, type-II
    neurons), atrophy, and gliosis in the head of the
    caudate and the putamen bilaterally, thus qualifying
    it as a subcortical dementia. However, moderate loss
    of neurons also occurs in layers 3, 5, and 6 of the
    cerebral cortex, making the clear differentiation
    between these two classes of dementia uncertain.

5. Patients with subcortical dementias are most likely to
    display symptoms characteristic of disordered limbic
    functioning: apathy and disorders of attention, mood,
    and memory. Cortical dementias, on the other hand,
    interrupt higher-order associative functioning, pro-
    ducing aphasia, agnosia, apraxia, and impaired ab-
    straction. Memory is impaired in both classes of
    dementia.

6. Depression is the most common psychiatric problem
    encountered among Huntington patients: most patients
    with HD feel depressed from time to time, whereas 40%
    suffer from a major depression at some point. De-
    pressed feelings are equally common among those at
    risk of developing HD as they wrestle with the uncer-
    tainties of their future: ie, how to plan for mar-
    riage, job, and children without knowing if they will
    develop this fatal illness. Finally, serious
    depression also seems to develop in some of these
    patients on a biological basis and such depressions
    may precede or follow the onset of neurological
    symptoms or dementia.
        Mr. K had coped successfully for 43 years with
    the uncertainty of his family history and then sudden-
    ly developed a major depression which responded only
    modestly to medication. This depression was most
    likely directly associated with his underlying bio-
    logical pathology. On the other hand, most presympto-
    matic HD patients who develop depression in reaction
    to their life's uncertainty have a pattern of depres-
    sion off and on for years.

7. Particularly dementia, depression, emotional lability,
    apathy, and anxiety but also mania, thought disorder,
    and other psychotic-like symptoms. Any of these symp-
    toms may appear months or years before the movement
    disorder. Moreover, many of these psychiatric presen-
    tations will respond to appropriate medication (eg,
    antidepressants for depression, antipsychotics for
    psychosis).

PEARLS:

1. Children whose father carries the HD gene are much
    more likely to develop symptoms at an early age than
    are those whose mother has the disease. The reason
    for this is unknown; it certainly flies in the face of
    traditional Mendelian genetics.

2. Once thought to be rare, Huntington's disease is now
    recognized as one of the most common autosomal dominant
    conditions.

3. Antidepressant medication is generally useful for the somatic symptoms of depression in HD patients (insomnia, anorexia) but of lesser use for the cognitive presentation (eg, sense of helplessness and hopelessness).

4. The psychiatric symptoms of the HD patient are generally more distressing to family members than are the neurological problems.

PITFALLS:

1. Don't focus on the neurological symptoms of HD to the exclusion of the psychiatric features - HD has one of the highest rates of suicide of any illness.

2. One must exercise special caution in prescribing antipsychotics to HD patients so as not to exacerbate the movement disorder with neuroleptic induced akathesias, dystonias, or dyskinesias.

TRIVIA:

1. Approximately 40% of the population in a small community on the shores of Lake Maracaibo, Venezuela either have HD or are at a 50% risk of developing it.

REFERENCES

1. Adams RD, Victor M: Principles of Neurology. New York, McGraw-Hill Book Co., 1985.
2. Bird SJ: Presymptomatic testing for Huntington's disease. JAMA 253:3286-3291, 1985.
3. Caine ED, Shoulson I: Psychiatric syndromes in Huntington's disease. Am J Psychiat 140:728-733, 1983.
4. Cummings JL, Benson F: Subcortical dementia: Review of an emerging concept. Arch Neurol 41:874-879, 1984.
5. Folstein SE, Franz ML, et al: Conduct disorder and affective disorder among the offspring of patients with Huntington's disease. Psychological Med 13:45-52, 1983.
6. Folstein SE, Phillips JA, et al: Huntington's Disease: Two families with differing clinical features show linkage to the G8 probe. Science 229:776-779, 1985.
7. Huber SJ, Paulson GW: The concept of subcortical dementia. Am J Psychiat 142:1312-1317, 1985.
8. Jeste DV, Wyatt RJ: Neuropsychiatric Movement Disorders. Washington, DC, Amer Psychiatric Press, 1984.
9. Gusella JF, Wexler NS, et al: A polymorphic DNA marker genetically linked to Huntington's disease. Nature 306:234-238, 1983.

CASE 26: A 36-year-old man has suffered from chronic
undifferentiated schizophrenia since he was 16 years old.
He has been in the State Hospital on five occasions and has
had innumerable other short (1-2 months) psychiatric
hospitalizations. He has just moved in with his brother's
family in Merry Dell, Utah - 150 miles away from the
nearest psychiatrist but just around the corner from your
family practice office. The brother, a longtime patient of
yours, asks you to care for him.
     He has been maintained on antipsychotic medication for
20 years: most recently 30 mg of Prolixin PO HS for the
past 5 years. His brother warns that without his medication, he can get "crazy." In fact, it has been a lack of
medication that has precipitated many of the past hospitalizations.
     You meet the patient. He is quiet, unsmiling, slow of
speech and movement, lucid, cooperative, non-psychotic, and
without complaint.

UNEASY OBSERVATION:

     The patient says he sees no reason for taking medica-
     tion and asks that it be stopped.

QUESTIONS:

1.   Would you stop his medication?

2.   What is the most serious risk of long-term antipsycho-
     tic use?

3.   Is this patient at risk for an acute dystonic reaction?

4.   Is the patient's lucid, non-psychotic presentation any
     guide to his current condition?

5.   What is the most common reason that schizophrenic
     patients stop their medication?

ANSWERS:

1.   Maybe. You would evaluate his condition and his past
      medication history and form a conclusion independent
      of the demands of either patient or family. "The past
      is the best predictor of the future" should be your
      primary guide. If you have irrefutable evidence (as
      opposed to "family rumor") that stopping medication in
      the past routinely resulted in decompensation, be
      reluctant to stop it (eg, a trial without medication
      perhaps every 5 years). Otherwise, chronic schizo-
      phrenics who are stable need a trial without meds
      about every 1-2 years.

2.   Tardive dyskinesia - involuntary, choreiform movements
      primarily of the tongue, lips, face, fingers, and
      hands that can appear months or years after the drugs
      were started. In some cases these movements are ir-
      reversible.

3.   No. Acute dystonic reactions typically occur during
      the first several days after antipsychotics are begun
      or after the dose has been significantly increased.

4.   Yes. A chronic schizophrenic patient who is without
      evidence of active psychosis is probably stable. Don't
      assume that there is a "beast" lurking inside the
      schizophrenic just waiting to get out if medication is
      stopped.

5.   Unpleasant medication side effects like akathesia,
      blurred vision, a Parkinson-like syndrome, and impo-
      tence. It behooves the physician to pay close atten-
      tion to complaints about side effects.

PEARLS:

1.   You will encounter schizophrenics in practice. About
      one third of the several million schizophrenics in the
      United States are treated by non-psychiatrists.

2.   The most effective course in the long-term treatment
      of many schizophrenics is to work closely with both
      the patient and his family.

3.   More than one half of chronic schizophrenics attempt
      suicide at some time. Antidepressant medication is an
      effective treatment with many of these patients.

4.   A therapy group which discusses the value and problems
      of medication is an effective way of encouraging medi-
      cation compliance among schizophrenics.

5.   Always try to maintain the <u>lowest</u> effective long-term
     dose of medication.

6.   Tardive dyskinesia is rapidly becoming the most common
     source of malpractice lawsuits against psychiatrists.

PITFALLS:

Screen the medication history obtained from either
the patient or his family carefully. Either may have
a vested interest in seeing the medication stopped or
continued, without appreciation for the patient's real
medication needs.

REFERENCES

1.   Diamond RJ: Enhancing medication use in schizophrenic
     patients. J Clin Psychiat 44:7-14, June, 1983.
2.   Hogan RP, Awad AG, Eastwood R: A self-report scale
     predictive of drug compliance in schizophrenics.
     Psycholo Med 13:177-183, 1983.
3.   Jeste DV, Wyatt RJ: Prevention and management of tar-
     dive dyskinesia. J Clin Psychiat 46:14-18, 1985.
4.   Johnson DAW: Antipsychotic medication: Clinical guide-
     lines for maintenance therapy. J Clin Psychiat 46:6-
     15, April, 1985.
5.   Kane JM: Compliance issues in outpatient treatment. J
     Clin Psychopharm 5:22S-27S, 1985.
6.   Kane JM: <u>Drug Maintenance Strategies in Schizophrenia</u>.
     Washington, DC, Amer Psychiatric Press, 1984.
7.   Roy A, Mazonson A, Pickar D: Attempted suicide in
     chronic schizophrenia. Brit J Psychiat 144:303-306,
     1984.
8.   Tomb DA: <u>Psychiatry for the House Officer</u>. Baltimore,
     Williams & Wilkins, 1984.
9.   Van Putten T: Why do schizophrenic patients refuse to
     take their drugs? Arch Gen Psychiat 31:67-72, 1974.

CASE 27: A 43-year-old white female came to the psychiatric outpatient department complaining of an overwhelming need to wash herself.

The patient began to wash her hands excessively in childhood. She remembers being ostracized by her grade school friends because of her insistence on cleanliness. In high school she avoided public rest rooms and was "forced to be a loner" because of her excessive fussiness and handwashing.

At present, her life is controlled by her fear of being soiled. She wakes in the morning dreading the need for a bowel movement and hopes that she can avoid one. If she defecates, she feels contaminated and needs to wipe herself at least ten times with two-ply soft toilet paper. Then she has to wash her hands until they feel clean. If she splashes soap or water anywhere while washing, she must then clean the sink, walls, faucets, carpet, or whatever else she suspects has been splashed. On the average she spends about two hours washing herself in the morning. (For months she has consumed a pint of whiskey each day to suppress the urge to defecate.)

In addition to the above behavior, she will take long showers after a bowel movement and repeatedly clean the perianal area. After the shower, she will carefully clean the walls while wearing rubber gloves. She frequently cleans the toilet with full-strength Lysol, and is careful to use separate clean rags for washing and rinsing. In an attempt to limit her cleaning, she has declared one toilet in the house off-limits to everyone but herself. She will handle her family's underwear only with gloves or other protection for her hands, washes the underwear with extra bleach and extra rinses, and insists that her husband empty the washer.

She is also obsessed with the fear of contamination by animal feces and will cross the street to avoid any stools on or near the sidewalk. When it rains, she is preoccupied with the thought that the rainwater is tainted with animal feces. If she gets her shoes wet, they are irreparably defiled and she then needs to throw them out. If she has to drive with contaminated shoes on, she insists that her husband wash the brake and gas pedals of the car.

She denies any obsessions or compulsions concerning urination or menstruation. However, she is presently having mid-cycle bleeding secondary to an apparent misuse of her oral contraceptives.

Her behavior has affected her life in other ways as well. At age 20, she saw her fiance's father picking his nose and thereafter "wanted nothing to do with him." She developed the need to shower after he greeted her and scrub the floors he had walked on. Three years ago, the patient developed a severe GI disturbance as a result of her attempts to prevent bowel movements. She would avoid a movement for about three weeks, then have an episode of explosive diarrhea.

This abnormal behavior has been present throughout two former marriages and has precipitated two divorces. Her third marriage is now at risk. (This threat to her marriage appears to be the reason she currently is seeking help.) Curiously, she had no difficulty delivering her two children or cleaning them as infants; however, she was unable to participate effectively in their toilet training.

Over the years, she has been in psychotherapy several times and has received a variety of medications including antipsychotics, minor tranquilizers, and antidepressants. Invariably, she has stopped treatment prematurely. Two years ago she was hospitalized, seemed to respond to a trial of lithium, but stopped that medication as well.

On presentation in the clinic, her mental status examination was unremarkable except for significant anxiety and mild, chronic feelings of depression. She is convinced that her problems stem from an episode of sexual molestation by her grandfather when she was six. Based on the presence of ego-dystonic obsessions and compulsions, the outpatient psychiatrist made a diagnosis of Obsessive Compulsive Disorder (DSM-III 300.00) (along with alcohol abuse and a probable mixture of personality disorders), and then wondered what to do next.

QUESTIONS:

1. Is there any hope for this woman? After all, she has been incapacitated to one degree or another since childhood.

2. Name the three common "classic" types of OCD.

3. What psychological treatments might help her?

4. Of what value are medications?

ANSWERS:

1. Yes. Obsessive Compulsive Disorder (OCD) has been extremely resistant to traditional psychodynamic forms of treatment. However, the use of behavioral techniques and medication in recent years has had much greater success.

2. <u>Washers</u> - 50% of patients; obsessed with a fear of contamination; they wash themselves and their surroundings excessively.
    <u>Checkers</u> - patients who have a certainty that they have forgotten, overlooked, or experienced something important which, if not checked on, will result in disaster.
    <u>Pure obsessionals</u> - 25% of patients; experience recurrent, intrusive, unwanted sexual or aggressive thoughts.

    Many patients are mixtures of these types. Most patients have both obsessions and compulsions (rituals) but a few have only obsessions (pure obsessionals).

3. <u>Behavior therapy</u>. Two techniques are of proven utility in many patients, particularly when used together:
    <u>Exposure</u> - the patient is exposed to the avoided situation <u>in vivo</u>. This technique is made as "real life" as possible (eg, the above patient might be asked to work in the hospital laundry room.)
    <u>Response prevention</u> - the compulsive behaviors are prevented (eg, the above patient might be denied access to a sink or to water).

    Combined, these two techniques have been shown to be effective with the majority of patients. However, they cannot be applied to the pure obsessionals who have no situations to avoid or rituals to modify.
    Besides behavioral therapy, support or encouragement is crucial if the patient is to remain in treatment.

4. <u>Antidepressants</u>, particularly clomipramine (not available in the U.S.) and possibly imipramine, benefit many patients. Depressed OCD patients are most likely to improve, thus it remains unresolved whether the effect of medication is primarily antiobsessional or antidepressant. However, antidepressants that are specific serotonin reuptake inhibitors (like clomipramine and fluoxetine) appear to be most effective, suggesting that they possess a unique antiobsessional effect.

On the other hand, a variety of medications have been found to be useful in individual cases (eg, MAO inhibitors, stimulants, alprazolam, pyridoxine, antipsychotics). A good rule of thumb is: if a drug other than an antidepressant is found to work, use it. The patient above responded to lithium during a previous hospitalization, so it was reinstated. With ample encouragement (pressure) from her husband, she stayed on the medication this time and was still improved at one year follow-up.

PEARLS:

1. Almost one half of all cases of OCD begin in childhood.

2. Most patients improve but are not "cured." Whether treated with medication or psychotherapy, many people continue to have low-level, nagging obsessional ideas and a desire to avoid situations or engage in rituals.

3. Severe obsessive compulsive illness is one of the last remaining indications for psychosurgery.

4. OCD sleep EEGs are a close, but not perfect, fit with those from depressed patients.

5. As many as 2% of the population may meet the criteria for OCD. Most do not seek treatment.

6. OCD is a chronic, remitting disorder.

7. Many "checkers" have a strict religious background.

8. Over half the patients with OCD develop a significant depression at some time.

PITFALLS:

1. Many patients with OCD present an irresistible lode of intrapsychic conflicts and symbolism to the psychodynamically inclined therapist. Some therapists just can't pass up the opportunity to do traditional, insight-oriented psychotherapy with these patients in spite of its ineffectiveness.

2. Some obsessional "directives" are so real and compelling to the patient that they can be mistaken by the examiner for auditory hallucinations ("voices") and the wrong diagnosis made. Make certain to differentiate voices the patient actually <u>hears</u> from thoughts (no matter how clear and forceful) that the patient <u>thinks</u>.

3.   The biggest problem in applying the behavioral tech-
     nique of exposure is that the patient may be too
     frightened to participate and thus drop out of treat-
     ment.   Careful attention to support and the develop-
     ment of rapport is essential.

REFERENCES

1.   Ananth J: Clomipramine in obsessive-compulsive dis-
     order: A review. Psychosomatics 24:723-727, 1983.
2.   Pies R: Distinguishing obsessional from psychotic
     phenomena. J Clin Psychopharmacol 4:345-347, 1984.
3.   Steketee G, Foa EB, Grayson JB: Recent advances in the
     behavioral treatment of obsessive-compulsives. Arch
     Gen Psychiatry 39:1365-1371, 1982.
4.   Turner SM, Jacob RG, et al: Fluoxetine treatment of
     obsessive-compulsive disorder. J Clin Psychopharmacol
     5:207-212, 1985.
5.   Turns DM: Epidemiology of phobic and obsessive-compul-
     sive disorders among adults. Amer J Psychotherapy
     34:360-370, 1985.
6.   Insel TR: New Findings in Obsessive-Compulsive Disorder.
     Washington, DC, American Psychiatric Press, 1984.
7.   Yaryura-Tobias JA, Neziroglu FA: Obsessive-Compulsive
     Disorder. New York, Marcel Dekker, 1983.

CASE 28: Mr. S, a 79-year-old man, stormed into the office with his 63-year-old wife in tow. Over the preceding several months he had been unable to "get it up" or "keep it up." When his internist asked him what he expected at 79, Mr. S became furious, prompting the current referral for a "sexual dysfunction neurosis."

Mr. S reported (forcefully) that he had always been sexually vigorous and certainly didn't need a psychiatrist to tell him "how to do it." He pointed to his "young wife" as proof of his virility. She, on the other hand, was reluctant to talk about such matters.

Until about 4 months ago he had sexual intercourse at least weekly, and sometimes twice each week. He found his recent failures (the first he had ever experienced) frustrating and wanted to get the problem solved.

His health had always been good; just mild hypertension for which he had taken hydrochlorothiazide for many years. His social life was satisfactory: he had recently (and finally) turned over his hardware business to his son and moved to a retirement community. He and his wife had several new friends and were enjoying their new environment.

PSYCHOSOCIAL CLUE:

Mrs. S assured the psychiatrist that things couldn't be better between herself and her husband.

QUESTIONS:

1.   Provide three synonymous names for his complaint.

2.   At 79, does Mr. S have any grounds for complaint?

3.   What physical systems are involved in potency?

4.   What should you do next?

5.   Explain Mr. S's problem.

6.   What are some physical ways to treat this condition?

ANSWERS:

1.   Impotence; erectile impotence; inhibited sexual excitement.

2.   Yes. Properly encouraged, most older people can stay sexually active well into their 80's. Impotence at age 79 is abnormal (although not uncommon).
     An older male can expect the following changes: (1) an erection will take longer to reach and will be softer, (2) an orgasm will be briefer and the force of semen ejection will decrease, and (3) the "refractory period" (time before another orgasm can be achieved) may be measured in days rather than minutes. These changes are presumably based on a gradual deterioration of the normal neurovascular mechanisms which maintain potency.

3.   Vascular: erection is produced by the two corpora cavernosa of the penis rapidly filling with blood. This blood comes from the internal iliac artery, through the internal pudendal artery, into the penile arteries, and finally through numerous arteriolar valves (polsters) into the corpora.
     Neural: Sensation from the penis passes through the pudendal nerves to produce either (1) a reflex erection through the nervi erigentes (ie, via a local, sacral parasympathetic motor arc) or (2) a considered erection by passing to the limbic system and cerebral cortex and then back through the nervi erigentes. Or, the impulse for erection may start directly in the cerebral cortex.
     Hormonal: Sexual desire, but not erection, is hormone dependent.

4.   Perform a careful history to look for the common medical and psychological causes of impotence.
     Psychogenic causes predominate at every age except the very old. Look for early morning erections, erections to stimuli other than the usual partner (eg, lover, erotic films), partial erections, obvious fears or psychological concerns around intercourse (eg, fear of having a heart attack), marital discord, or lack of adequate sexual desire.
     Organic causes are multiple and include drugs (diuretics and antihypertensives, anticholinergics, alcohol, major tranquilizers, antidepressants, etc), vascular impairment (eg, localized atherosclerotic blockage, microvascular disease associated with diabetes, etc), neural impairment (radical pelvic surgery which disrupts the nervi erigentes, diabetic

peripheral neuropathy, etc), and endocrinological (hypogonadism, hyperprolactinemia, etc). However, most organic dysfunction has an associated secondary overlay of psychogenic impairment. Moreover, psychological and organic factors are often additive and can impair potency together when neither would alone.

In addition to suggestive history, several tests help in the differentiation of organic from functional causes: fasting glucose and glucose tolerance tests, serum testosterone, nocturnal penile tumescence sleep studies (NPT - nighttime erections during REM sleep are very suggestive of a psychological etiology), a good physical exam including femoral and lower limb pulses, arteriography of the internal pudendal artery, penile blood pressure measurements. None of these tests are foolproof and thus should be interpreted with caution.

Mr. S had a normal (for age) FG and GTT as well as clear morning erection by history.

5.   His impotence was probably primarily psychogenic. Although he thought of himself as virile (but did he "protest too much"?), he suddenly was living in a new environment surrounded by the elderly, he no longer was the boss of a small company, and his wife was quickly developing new interests and new friends and was clearly not too worried about his failing potency ("Our relationship couldn't be better"). Without his former supports and the encouragement of his wife, his performance was faltering. Moreover, because of his age and chronic mild hypertension, his organic capabilities were probably marginal and did not require too great of a psychological stress to precipitate a decline.

After two sessions alone with the psychiatrist, Mr. S returned to his previous level of functioning. He was given a chance to voice his general concerns about his new living situation and received abundant assurance that the impotence was probably transitory. Equally important, his wife was instructed as to the importance of her continued direct, if subtle, encouragement of his sexual efforts.

6.   Psychogenic impotence should generally be treated by psychological means. Improved physical health, medication modification, and treatment of specific medical conditions will occasionally improve organic impotence. Psychological techniques should be applied to all cases.

Unfortunately, many organic causes are irreversible. For these patients, surgical implantation of semirigid Silastic rods or an inflatable penile prosthesis may help. However, these techniques are controversial and may produce an unsatisfactory result.

PEARLS:

1.   Most impotence in young men is psychological.

2.   The older the patient, the more likely it is that his impotence is organic.

3.   The sense of "orgasm" in the human male is merely due to the rhythmic contraction of the bulbocavernosus and ischiocavernosus muscles.

4.   Patients who are slow to erect but who ejaculate "on time" may thus experience functional premature ejaculation.

5.   Several studies of impotent men suggest that a majority of those with "organic" impotence respond to psychotherapy.

6.   Once discontinued, the ability to perform sexually is often hard for the elderly male to regain ("If you don't use it, you lose it").

7.   NPT occasionally occurs with an organic etiology just as lack of nighttime tumescence does not rule out a psychological cause.

8.   The most crucial contribution of healthy sexuality to emotional health in old age is its capacity to enhance intimacy.

PITFALLS:

Do not permit your discomfort with old age sexuality to cause you to covertly or overtly discourage your older patient from participating in healthy sex. One major reason for sexual inactivity among the elderly is social pressure and expectations (although physical problems and lack of a partner play important roles as well).

REFERENCES

1. Bancroft J, Wu FC: Erectile impotence. Brit Med J
    290:1566-1568, 1985.
2. Fallon B, Rosenberg S, Culp DA: Long-term followup in
    patients with an inflatable penile prosthesis. J Urol
    132:270-271, 1984.
3. Finkle AL: Sexual psychodynamics of aging: Urologic
    perspectives. J Amer Geriat Soc 25:393-395, 1977.
4. Hollander JB, Diokno AC: Success with penile prosthesis
    from patient's viewpoint. Urol 23:141-143, 1984.
5. Karacan I: Nocturnal penile tumescence as a biologic
    marker in assessing erectile dysfunction. Psychosom
    23:350-360, 1982.
6. Silber SJ: Impotence. Adv Int Med 30:359-385, 1984.
7. Spark RF, White RA, Connolly PB. Impotence is not
    always psychogenic. JAMA 243:750-755, 1980.
8. Wagner G, Green R: Impotence: Physiological, Psycho-
    logical, Surgical Diagnosis and Treatment. New York,
    Plenum Press, 1981.
9. Wasserman MD, Pollak CP, et al: The differential diag-
    nosis of impotence. JAMA 243:2038-2042, 1980.

CASE 29: Mrs. W, an 86-year-old, widowed, Dutch immigrant, is brought to the emergency room by her daughter who complains, "My mother has gone crazy." The history apparently began about two months ago when Mrs. W was living in Los Angeles with her 48-year-old, single son. One of them, it is unclear which, began to believe that there were ghosts in the apartment and their lives were in danger if they stayed. The other began to share the belief and they shortly packed what belongings would fit into the car and left. They traveled around the Southwest for six weeks, living in the car and eventually running out of money. To their dismay, they found that wherever they went the ghosts were present. Mrs. W began hearing voices. She was told, "We will never let you go," "We are going to get you with steam and electricity," "You are the boss of America," "You are going to be the mother of the Anti-Christ," "You are hypnotized," and "You are to marry the Pope."

The daughter became aware of this trouble after receiving a few cryptic phone calls, but her mother and brother never remained in one place long enough for her to locate them. They finally came to the attention of Las Vegas police and were detained long enough for the daughter to fly in. She flew her mother home and took her directly to the hospital, leaving her brother to fend for himself.

Mrs. W presented with clear sensorium, good memory, bright and pleasant affect, and no evidence of depression. Her thoughts were clear and goal directed, yet centered around "the ghosts." They had followed her to the hospital and she continued to hear their voices.

HISTORICAL CLUE:

Past history was negative for mental illness of any type. She had been happy, pleasant and hard-working, not retiring from her duties as a housekeeper until age 77. She had always enjoyed good health and did not use alcohol or medication of any type.

QUESTIONS:

1. What is the diagnosis?

2. What is it called when two people share delusional beliefs?

3. Why do you suppose the ghosts threatened her with steam and electricity?

4. Should she have her ears examined?

5. What treatment would you recommend?

ANSWERS:

1. This type of problem has been known and written about
    for decades, yet arguments continue over diagnostic
    terminology. The patient presents neither organic nor
    affective components. The problem then is one of
    paranoid delusions and auditory hallucinations with
    onset at age 86. This condition has been variously
    called paraphrenia, late paraphrenia, late-onset psy-
    chosis, involutional paranoia, late-life schizophrenia,
    senile schizophrenia, and atypical paranoid disorder.
    (The DSM-III term "shared paranoid disorder" would be
    a secondary diagnosis in this case, as well - see
    answer #2.) The boundaries of this disorder and its
    differentiation from similar disorders, such as para-
    noid personality and paranoid schizophrenia, is un-
    clear. The major differentiation is an arbitrary one
    in most classification schemes - age (45 y/o and over
    in DSM-III). Such "late-onset" patients generally do
    not show marked formal thought disorder (such as loose
    associations or incoherence), deterioration with time,
    or prominent hallucinations. In DSM-III terms, Mrs.
    W's diagnosis would be Atypical Paranoid Disorder
    (DSM-III 297.90) - the atypical feature being the
    auditory hallucinations.
        This disorder occurs most commonly between ages
    60 and 80 in women who are single and socially isola-
    ted. The most common premorbid personalities are
    paranoid and schizoid.
        The delusions encountered are commonly simple
    alternative explanations for real-life events. These
    are usually less bizarre and esoteric than those seen
    in young schizophrenics. Themes often revolve around
    domestic issues, possessions, sexual virtue, or, per-
    sonal identity. Common examples would be: "Someone is
    stealing my mail," "People break into my garage every
    night and take things," "The neighbors have installed
    a telescope facing my bedroom and they look in day and
    night," or "My ex-husband pumps gas into my house to
    knock me out."

2. The term "folie a deux" has been updated in the DSM-
    III to "shared paranoid disorder," and refers to a
    paranoid delusional system that develops between two
    people. Commonly, one person is dominant with more
    fixed delusions and the other more suggestible or
    dependent. It is likely that Mrs. W's son was dominant
    and more chronically paranoid, but this was never
    proven. The condition is rare and occurs most fre-
    quently in women and in those who live together in a
    close existence that is rather isolated from the out-
    side world.

3. Why people elaborate certain delusional beliefs has
    long been the subject of psychodynamic speculation.
    Although uncertain, some generalizations seem to hold.
    Delusional content appears to be determined in part by
    cultural and commonly held beliefs. For instance,
    many delusional American Christians believe themselves
    to be Christ. Delusional Oriental Buddhists do not.
    Paranoid delusions often center around the fears or
    enemies of a society. It would be unusual today but
    common in years long past for one to develop delusions
    centering around Napoleon. Today's enemies are more
    commonly the Mafia, Communists, or other persons of
    fear or influence. Religious and scientific themes
    are common - possibly because they incorporate themes
    of the unknown, the world that can't be seen, subtle
    influences, or unlimited power. Today people are
    commonly delusional about nuclear power, computers,
    and space travel. Fears of steam and electricity
    suggest similar themes from an era long past, the
    turn-of-the-century era of Mrs. W's childhood.

4. Definitely, and her eyes, too. Of patients with
    late-onset paranoid disorder, 40% have moderate to
    severe hearing loss, and visual impairment is almost
    as common. Such sensory losses are significant etio-
    logical factors in the late-life paranoias. As one's
    contact with the "real world" diminishes through com-
    promised vision or hearing (or even compromised taste,
    smell, or touch) they may begin to interpret distorted
    images or muddled sounds as referring to themselves in
    uncomplimentary or sinister ways. Social isolation is
    felt to have a similar impact - limiting normal social
    cues necessary to appropriately interpret the
    environment.

5. The mainstay of treatment in this group is neuroleptic
    medication. Over 85% of those who receive adequate
    treatment have total and sustained remission of their
    psychotic symptoms. The most commonly used
    neuroleptics in this group are haloperidol, thiothixene,
    and thioridazine.
        General measures that would apply to most such
    patients include establishing a stable, safe, friendly
    environment; correction of sensory losses (see answer
    #4); and good nutrition (Mrs. W had eaten nothing but
    bread and milk for six weeks). Hospitalization is
    often necessary in those without close family super-
    vision. Post (1982) has established the most optimis-
    tic prognostic factors to be (1) rapid improvement on
    medication, (2) a stable marriage, (3) early age of
    onset, (4) adherence to maintenance medication, and
    (5) development of insight.

PEARLS:

1. It is estimated that patients with late-life psychosis account for about 10% of geriatric psychiatry admissions, making it one of the most commonly encountered mental problems of the elderly.

2. In a recent study, mean age of onset was 70.

3. This disorder is much more common in women than men (7:1).

4. In DSM-III terms, the feature that usually distinguishes "typical" from "atypical" paranoid disorder in the elderly is the presence or absence of hallucinations. This distinction seems artificial and may be eliminated in future diagnostic schemes.

5. Psychotropic medication given to paranoid patients should be in liquid form. In one study, 70% of the tablets given to paranoid patients were never taken.

6. Both the deaf and blind show an increased incidence of paranoia.

7. Most patients with late-life paranoia either have no children or limited contact with their children.

PITFALLS:

1. The above terms (paraphrenia, late-life psychosis, etc - see answer #1) do not refer to chronic schizophrenics whose illness has continued into old age.

2. Organic mental disorders and affective disorders can resemble late-life paranoia.

TRIVIA:

1. The term "paranoia" is derived from the Greek roots "para," meaning beside, and "nous," meaning mind. The paranoid were literally beside their right minds.

2. The term "paraphrenia" dates back to the early 19th century and is a condensation of "paranoia" and "schizophrenia."

REFERENCES

1. American Psychiatric Association Task Force on Nomenclature and Statistics: Diagnostic and Statistical Manual of Mental Disorders, 3rd ed. (DSM-III). Amer. Psychiatric Association, Washington, DC, 1980.
2. Leuchter AF: Assessment and treatment of the late-onset psychoses. Hosp Comm Psychiatry 36:815-18, 1985.
3. Leuchter AF, Spar JE: The late-onset psychoses: Clinical and diagnostic features. J Nerv Ment Dis 173:488-494, 1985.
4. Post F: The Psychiatry of Late Life, Boston, Blackwell Scientific Pub, 1982.
5. Verwoerdt A: Clinical Geropsychiatry. 2nd ed., Baltimore, Williams & Wilkins, 1981.

CASE 30: Jerry, a 35-year-old white male, is brought to the emergency room by the police. He is an inmate at the nearby state prison and twenty minutes before had been cut down from the bars of his cell after he had tried to hang himself.

Although initially delirious secondary to anoxia suffered during his suicide attempt, he rapidly became lucid and gave the following history. He had spent, on and off, a total of 13 years in prison for innumerable burglaries and several armed robberies and had six more years left in his current sentence. He didn't like prison and occasionally became badly depressed for days or weeks at a time as he contemplated his situation. Today, for reasons he didn't understand, things looked particularly black. He had tried to change his mood with some "downers" illicitly obtained from another prisoner but they were of no help. In a fit of hopelessness, he rolled his shirt, wrapped it around a bar, and jumped from a book placed on end. He then only remembers struggling to free himself unsuccessfully.

His record describes a 9th grade education and criminal activity since his early teens. Most of his arrests have been for thefts of one kind or another. There is little history of assaults or violent behavior. Apparently he has also used a variety of drugs over the years, although there is no suggestion of addiction to a single substance. The diagnosis seen repeatedly in his prison record is antisocial personality disorder.

After he has recovered from his delirium, he chats freely and openly. He is honest about his past, seems chagrined at his illegal behavior, convincingly describes serious depressive feelings, and wishes his life had turned out otherwise. He is warm, friendly, humorous, and thoroughly likeable. The house officer silently questions the propriety of "labeling" such an engaging human being with antisocial personality disorder and is mildly upset as the police brusquely usher the prisoner from the emergency room after his physical status has stabilized.

ENVIRONMENTAL CLUE:

As the house officer is berating the attending psychiatrist for his tendency to affix pejorative diagnoses to people, the nurse enters the room to inform the resident that two vials of injectable diazepam are missing from the crash cart in the hall.

QUESTIONS:

1. Name two approximate synonyms for "antisocial person-
    ality disorder."

2. Did this patient have antisocial PD?

3. Was he depressed?

4. Does he represent a suicide risk?

5. What happened to the diazepam?

ANSWERS:

1. So̲c̲i̲o̲p̲a̲t̲h̲y̲ (sociopath); p̲s̲y̲c̲h̲o̲p̲a̲t̲h̲y̲ (psychopath).
   These are older terms, still used by some professionals
   today, which refer roughly to the same population.

2. Yes. This diagnosis is now based almost exclusively
   on the presence of antisocial b̲e̲h̲a̲v̲i̲o̲r̲. The individual
   must (1) have displayed significant antisocial behavior
   before the age of 15 (eg, truancy, delinquency, thefts,
   vandalism, lying, fighting, substance abuse) and (2)
   have been actively engaged in antisocial behavior
   since adulthood (eg, theft, violence, poor work history, unstable interpersonal relationships, unpaid
   debts, recklessness, impulsiveness). The patient
   above easily fulfilled the requirements in both categories.
      Although this is the most specific and diagnos-
   tically reliable of the personality disorders, it is
   criticized in two areas. First, many antisocial
   adults showed little childhood criminality yet probably should receive the diagnosis as adults. Second,
   the current classification makes no mention of the
   psychological accompaniments of this behavior: guilt-
   lessness, an inability to form close relationships, a
   drive for excitement, etc. Thus, the diagnosis of
   antisocial PD is likely to be revised in the future.

3. Probably. Patients with antisocial PD become depressed
   with a greater frequency than the general public. In
   part this reflects the unpleasant circumstances their
   behavior forces upon them (eg, prison), but they also
   apparently have a higher incidence of "endogenous"
   depression and depression associated with substance
   abuse.
      However, as was the case with this patient, many
   depressive episodes are brief and reactive and reflect
   the underlying impulsiveness common to these individuals. Jerry was chatting and joking two hours after
   almost killing himself - probably in response to the
   pleasant change from the prison environment.

4. Yes. The impulsiveness of these people, coupled with
   frequent substance abuse, put them at increased risk
   of suicide.

5. Jerry took it (for later sale among the prison
   inmates); the ER called ahead and the vials were found
   wrapped in the shirt Jerry had tried to hang himself
   with. He impulsively grabbed the drugs even though,
   with a little reflection, he would have realized that

they would be found during the required search when he
re-entered the prison.

PEARLS:

1.   Three percent of men have antisocial PD (M:F = 5-10:1).

2.   A major adoption study (Mednick et al, 1984) concludes
      that there is a "biological predisposition" towards
      criminality passed from criminal parents to their off-
      spring.   In other words, some criminal behavior
      appears to have biological roots.

3.   Alcoholics are more likely to be sociopaths and socio-
      paths are more likely to be alcoholics, but the two
      conditions don't seem to be genetically related.

4.   Impulsive, violent behavior has been correlated with a
      low level of CSF 5-hydroxyindoleacetic acid (5-HIAA,
      the major metabolite of serotonin).

5.   In spite of the points above, criminality and antisoc-
      ial personality disorder are most strongly correlated
      with unstable, unhappy childhood environments, not
      biology.

6.   Approximately 50% of inmates in state prisons meet the
      diagnostic criteria for antisocial personality dis-
      order.   The most common reason the criteria are not
      met is a lack of early juvenile criminality.

PITFALLS:

1.   Be aware that a person with antisocial personality
      disorder can suffer from depression, anxiety, grief,
      joy, or any other human emotion or psychiatric dis-
      order - their complaints and symptoms are not always
      an effort to "con" you.

2.   On the other hand, these individuals will frequently
      mislead people in their own self-interest.   ("Let the
      buyer beware.")

TRIVIA:

      Sociopaths are more likely than other individuals to
      be ambidextrous.

REFERENCES

1. Bohman M, Cloninger R, et al: Predisposition to petty criminality in Swedish adoptees. Arch Gen Psychiatry 39:1233-1241, 1982.
2. Hare RD: Diagnosis of antisocial personality disorder in two prison populations. Am J Psychiatry 140:887-890, 1983.
3. Linnoila M, Virkkunen M, et al: Low cerebrospinal fluid 5-hydroxyindoleacetic acid concentration differentiates impulsive from nonimpulsive violent behavior. Life Sciences 33:2609-2614, 1983.
4. Mednick SA, Gabrielli WF, Hutchings B: Genetic influences in criminal convictions: Evidence from an adoption cohort. Science 224:891-894, 1984.
5. Reid WH: The antisocial personality: A review. Hosp and Comm Psychiatry 36:831-837, 1985.
6. Standage KF: Observations on the handedness preferences of patients with personality disorders. Brit J Psychiat 142:575-578, 1983.
7. Vaillant GE: Natural history of male alcoholism. V. Is alcoholism the cart or the horse to sociopathy? Brit J Addiction 78:317-326, 1983.

<u>CASE 31</u>: A 20-year-old man arrives for his first appointment looking sullen and mildly angry. He is superficially polite but appears reluctant to see you.

After a minute or two of introductions, you ask why he made the appointment. He responds initially with silence, and then states: "I've got no problem - my mother made me come. I live at home while I go to college but Mom is on my back all the time. She doesn't like my friends and says I need to do something about them - like see you."

You say "hum," and then wait. After a brief moment of silence, he blurts out: "I'm gay, and my mother just found out. She wants me to do something about it."

He then tells you "the whole story." He has been gay as long as he can remember. He always felt very close to his childhood boyfriends and had many homosexual encounters as a teenager. Girls have been "just friends," and not very close ones at that. He has never experienced any sexual attraction to females, has trouble imagining what it would be like, and finds the whole topic mildly disgusting. Being gay is "just the way I am." Since entering college, he has become even more sexually active, but has usually restricted that activity to bars, dorm rooms, and friends' apartments. However, last week his mother found him in his bed at home with a boyfriend and "freaked out." She insisted that he see a psychiatrist right away.

After he has completed his tale, you ask him again why he has come to see you. He replies: "I don't know - I guess I'll leave." Then he stands up and walks out.

OBSERVATIONAL CLUE:

An hour later his mother calls to ask why you refused to treat her son. She is furious and accuses you, and psychiatrists in general, of being homosexual.

QUESTIONS:

1. What is your diagnosis?

2. What causes this "non-condition?"

3. Are these people "moral monsters?"

4. Is this patient's lack of close female friends signifigant?

5. Is this man treatable?

ANSWERS:

1. No diagnosis. With DSM-III, the American Psychiatric Association made a much disputed, politically motivated decision to delete homosexuality from classification as a psychiatric disorder, even though a number of parallel conditions characterized primarily by arousal to "deviant" stimuli remain diagnosable.

    However, one related condition remains: if a person with a homosexual orientation is distressed by his (or her) condition, the diagnosis of ego-dystonic homosexuality can be made. This represents a small minority of all individuals with a same-sex orientation. (The patient above clearly was comfortable with his homosexuality and thus deserved no diagnosis. His mother, however, was very invested in seeing him get "help" - parents, the public, and society often view homosexuality as an aberration that should be treated, or punished.)

2. The cause(s) of homosexuality is (are) unknown. As might be expected, however, such an emotionally loaded condition has no shortage of proposed etiologies, from constitutional weakness to an "act of God." The three most trumpeted causes probably are:

    (1) Parental child rearing practices (the classic psychoanalytic view) - specifically, a strong or protective mother with whom the person can identify and an absent or cruel father who cannot serve as a model. Unfortunately, this pattern is not particularly prevalent among the parents of homosexuals, raising doubts about the theory.

    (2) Behavioral conditioning - early experiences with erotic, same-sex activities are supposed to condition a child to enjoy homosexual activities. However, many homosexuals recall arousal to homosexual ideas long before any experiences, bringing into question the primacy of conditioning.

    (3) Biological roots - Recent endocrinological evidence points to abnormalities of sexual differentiation among homosexuals which may reflect prenatal influences. These findings remain controversial.

3. Certainly not. Save for the sexual realm, homosexuals behave much like everyone else. In fact, one of the reasons for "declassifying" homosexuality was to help

remove the stigma from the condition. In certain communities, the prejudice against them can be crippling.

4. Not particularly. Some male homosexuals tend to be uneasy around women but many have close female friends. However, there does seem to be a stonger tendency for female homosexuals to avoid or dislike men. There is no generally accepted explanation for either of these observations.

5. Probably not. He is comfortable with his sexual orientation and doesn't see himself as a patient. However, if he wished to shift to a heterosexual orientation (for whatever reason - usually social pressure), effective treatment may be available.

    Although traditional psychodynamic psychotherapy is not effective in changing sexual orientation, some new behavioral methods work with many individuals. The trick is to treat specific issues separately: apply methods to decrease deviant arousal (eg, aversion therapy), <u>and</u> other methods to increase heterosexual arousal, <u>and</u> other methods to teach heterosocial skills, if needed. Treating one of these areas without addressing the others is usually ineffective. (Thus, the male homosexual who loses his interest in men does not immediately become interested in women.)

PEARLS:

1. Some male homosexuals are extraordinarily promiscuous, having several hundred partners in a year. Lesbians, on the other hand, are more likely to maintain a lasting relationship with one individual.

2. The majority of very effeminate boys become adult homosexuals and/or develop gender identity problems. The majority of female homosexuals were very tomboyish as children. These observations are felt by some experts to suggest a biological etiology for homosexuality.

3. Homosexuality is found in about equal numbers in all cultures studied.

4. Up to 30% of males and 20% of females have been aroused to the point of orgasm by a member of the same sex at some time since adolescence; 10% of males and 3-5% of women are primarily homosexual.

5. Although homosexuals have a much higher incidence of gender identity confusion than the general population, most male homosexuals feel like men and most lesbians feel feminine.

6. A one-time or even extensive homosexual experience forced on a child does not lead to homosexuality.

7. The prenatal hormonal environment (particularly levels of prenatal androgens) seems to play a central role in both adult gender identity and sexual object choice. However, the details are yet to be worked out.

8. A potential "lab test" for homosexuality is a female-like rise in serum luteinizing hormone to an estrogen challenge (see Gladue, 1984), although these results need replication (see Baum, 1985). This response is felt by some to reflect the basic biological nature of the condition.

PITFALLS:

Homosexuals are just people. To treat them otherwise is to do your patients a disservice. The goal of any psychological treatment for those comfortable with their homosexuality should probably be to improve their interpersonal relationships rather than to change their sexual orientation.

REFERENCES

1. Baum MJ, Carroll RS, et al: Neuroendocrine response to estrogen and sexual orientation. Science 230:960-961, 1985.

2. Gladue BA, Green R, Hellman RE: Neuroendocrine response to estrogen and sexual orientation. Science 225:1496-1499, 1984.

3. Goodman RE: Biology of sexuality. Brit J Psychiat 143:216-220, 1983.

4. Green R: Gender identity in childhood and later sexual orientation. Am J Psychiat 142:339-341, 1985.

5. Maccoby EE, Jacklin CN: The Psychology of Sex Differences. Stanford, CA, Stanford Univ Pr, 1974.

6. Saghir MT, Robins E: Male & Female Homosexuality. Baltimore, Williams & Wilkins, 1973.

7. Spence JT, Helmreich RL: Masculinity & Femininity. Austin, TX, Univ Texas Pr, 1978.

8. Stoller RJ, Herdt GH: Theories of origins of male homosexuality. Arch Gen Psychiat 42:399-404, 1985.

9. West DJ: Homosexuality and lesbianism. Brit J Psychiat 143:221-226, 1983.

THE NEVER-ENDING STORY

CASE 32:   You have been taking care of a 23-year-old schizophrenic patient since he was 16 years old. During that
time he has had 11 psychiatric hospitalizations, some
lasting as long as 4-5 months. Although thoroughly
psychotic at the time of each readmission, he generally has
improved enough by the end of these hospital stays for you
to be hopeful about his prognosis. Unfortunately, however,
try what you may, he then stumbles along for a few weeks or
months and finally relapses.

OBSERVATIONAL CLUES:

1.   Even though you have treated him for 7 years and
     through 11 hospitalizations, your patient still
     is moderately uncooperative, frequently misses
     appointments, and is unwilling to see himself as
     mentally ill.
2.   You hear from his distraught mother as much as you
     hear from him.

QUESTIONS:

1.   In evaluating this case afresh, what is the first
     thing you should do?

2.   What is the expected course of illness in schizophren-
     ia?

3.   Name four critical factors influencing the tendency to
     relapse.

4.   What are the early signs of a relapse?

5.   What should you do if a relapse is imminent?

ANSWERS:

1. Reconfirm the diagnosis. Certainly, anytime psychosis is interspersed with periods of fairly normal functioning, a chronic affective disorder should be considered. (However, this patient's clinical picture was classically schizophrenic and he had several relatives also similarly afflicted.)

2. It was once thought that schizophrenia pursued a chronic downhill course but it is now recognized that most patients are ill only intermittently. Whether this represents a basic change in the illness or is a reflection of modern treatment methods is not known, but the "young adult chronic" patient of today can expect to spend the majority of his time in outpatient settings and on the fringes of psychosis rather than being locked in state hospitals for long periods. (Thus, this patient's presentation is typical of many of today's schizophrenic patients.)

3. Maintenance medication. Low- to moderate-level antipsychotic medication is essential in maintaining a remission. Although a few patients will do well without it, we cannot yet reliably identify those individuals and thus need to treat the majority of patients with low-level antipsychotics for long periods. (All too many of these patients, such as the individual in this case, fail to appreciate their need for medication and thus take their medication unreliably. There was good evidence that several of this patient's rehospitalizations were precipitated by his voluntarily stopping his meds.)

    Life stress. Young schizophrenics are particularly sensitive to environmental stress and decompensate if too many demands are placed on them. Thus, an essential part of long-term treatment involves helping them develop a life style which minimizes stresses to which they may be particularly vulnerable (eg, finding an understanding and nondemanding boss, going to school part-time, working in a solitary and relaxed setting, etc). (This patient was under great family pressure to "make something of himself" and the therapist was continually discouraging the mother from pushing her son into a job as soon as he was released from the hospital.)

    Expressed emotion. This refers to family members who are overly "emotional" towards the patient: either hypercritical and too demanding or protective and over-invested (or, frequently, both). Some close relatives find it very hard to maintain a healthy objectivity toward the patient and continually involve themselves in his affairs. Schizophrenic patients appear to be particularly sensitive to such relentless "stirring the pot" by their close family members and quickly decompensate when living in such a "hot house" atmosphere. Encourage healthy family involvement but deal with excessive "expressed emotion" through family therapy.

The biology of the illness. Schizophrenics and their illnesses are not all alike. Some respond to our ministrations; others don't. The difference lies in the inherent nature of the disease in the individual patient. We don't yet understand the origin of these differences (we presume they are biological) but they play a major role in determining who relapses and who doesn't.

4.   They vary from patient to patient, yet over 90% of patients will have one or more of the following symptoms early in their decompensation: onset of hallucinations, increased suspiciousness, insomnia or fractured sleep, anxiety, and confused thinking. Patients are likely to repeat their pattern of decompensation in subsequent breakdowns.

5.   Reevaluate the patient's situation to identify key stressors and try to correct them. Increase a low maintenance medication dosage to acute levels until symptoms abate. Rapid pharmacologic intervention during the prodromal phase can often abort a developing psychotic episode.

PEARLS:

1.   Schizophrenia was once known as Dementia Praecox because it was felt to take a progressive downhill course, ending in dementia at an early age. That is no longer true.

2.   Patients on maintenance medication can tolerate much greater stress than they can without it. However, major stress will break through even the most vigorous medication schedule.

3.   Schizophrenia may be thought of as the patient having a "vulnerability" to a schizophrenic, psychotic state.

4. Because of the changing nature of schizophrenia, long-
    term treatment plans should focus on outpatient care
    and particularly on addressing the educational, social,
    and vocational needs of these patients.

5. The new "young adult chronic schizophrenic" differs
    from the older schizophrenic population not only in
    being less continuously psychotic but also in being
    more attention-seeking, help-rejecting, drug-abusing,
    promiscuous, and rootless. In other words, they are
    no less difficult to treat.

PITFALLS:

Don't fall into the trap of thinking of these patients
as "schizophrenics," as opposed to "people suffering
from schizophrenia." That is, we may not be talking
about a fixed, unalterable condition but rather about
a disease state.

REFERENCES

1. Barrowclough C, Tarrier N: Psychosocial interventions
    with families and their effects on the course of
    schizophrenia: A review. Psychol Med 14:629-642, 1984.
2. Doane JA, Falloon IRH, et al: Parental affective style
    and the treatment of schizophrenia. Arch Gen Psychiat
    42:34-42, 1985.
3. Gruen R, Baron M: Stressful life events and schizo-
    phrenia. Neuropsychobiology 12:206-208, 1984.
4. Heinrichs DW, Carpenter WT: Prospective study of pro-
    dromal symptoms in schizophrenic relapse. Am J Psychiat
    142:371-373, 1985.
5. Leff J, Kuipers L, et al: A controlled trial of social
    intervention in the families of schizophrenic patients.
    Brit J Psychiat 146:594-600, 1985.
6. Pepper B: The young adult chronic patient: Population
    overview. J Clin Psychopharm 5:3S-7S, 1985.
7. Snyder S: Phenomenology and treatment of the young
    adult chronic patient: A review. J Operational Psychiat
    16:32-36, 1985.
8. Zubin J, Magaziner J, Steinhauer SR: The metamorphosis
    of schizophrenia: From chronicity to vulnerability.
    Psychol Med 13:551-571, 1983.

CASE 33: A 27-year-old Hispanic graduate student presents with a chief complaint of depression. The problem began about three weeks ago and seemed related to the news that his evening job was being phased out. He reports that this was the third problem to befall him in as many months. "It started with fall quarter. I never really caught up in Statistics after missing a week with the flu, but I hadn't expected to get a "D" and have to repeat the course. Then about six weeks ago I found out my wife was pregnant. I tried to act happy for her but I wasn't. We already have three and are just barely making it financially. I was holding up pretty good until I heard about the job. I started crying right in front of the boss. I've just been hopeless ever since. I only go to school about half of the time - I don't like to be around anybody."

Further examination reveals no past or family history of depression and no apparent thought or personality disorder.

HISTORICAL CLUE:

> He denies anorexia, low energy, difficulty concentrating, suicide thoughts, or excessive guilt. A mild insomnia, characterized by difficulty falling to sleep, is present 3 or 4 nights a week.

QUESTIONS:

1. What is the diagnosis?

2. Of what value is the information provided in the clue?

3. Which would you prescribe - a tricyclic antidepressant or MAO inhibitor?

4. What diagnosis would apply if he had reacted to these problems with a modest depression and shown no impairment in school or social functioning?

5. What is the prognosis?

ANSWERS:

1. Adjustment disorder with depressed mood (DSM-III, 309.00). This diagnostic category indicates that life stress accompanies a depression which is less severe than a major depression but sufficient to impair functioning. In simple terms adjustment disorders are pathological responses to "bad luck." The maladaptive response may take the form of impaired social or occupational functioning, as in this case, or an excessive reaction to a stress. Symptoms vary, with depression, anxiety or anger predominating. Conduct disturbance is common in adolescence and physical symptoms common in children and the elderly.

    Stressors may be single (loss of job), multiple (as in this case), recurrent (seasonal business stresses), or continuous (chronic illness) and can involve individuals, families, or whole communities (as in natural disasters). Adjustment disorders are often associated with the stresses accompanying various life developmental stages such as starting school, marriage or retirement. In an adjustment disorder, life stress has disclosed an area of vulnerability in a person who is generally otherwise well adjusted.

2. This information essentially rules out major depression as the diagnosis. (It is possible that in certain individuals similar stresses could precipitate a major depression.) This distinction is important since it influences both treatment and prognosis.

3. Neither. There is nothing in the history or presentation to suggest that antidepressant medication is indicated. The patient may return to his previous level of functioning regardless of your treatment (see question 5). However, his improvement might be hastened and his ability to cope with future stresses fortified through psychotherapy. Also, therapy groups composed of persons who have undergone similar stresses may be beneficial. If the insomnia is problematic he may benefit from an occasional bedtime benzodiazepine.

4. Symptoms of a modest depression under these circumstances seem understandable and not outside the bounds of what might be considered normal. If this were his response and functioning was not impaired the diagnosis of adjustment disorder would not apply. The "V Codes" of DSM-III include conditions not attribu-

table to a mental disorder and are appropriately used to acknowledge the life problems of "normal" individuals who appear to cope adequately. Such distinctions are sometimes difficult and evade exact definition, yet under these circumstances the diagnoses "life circumstance problem" (DSM-III, V62.89), "academic problem" (V62.30), or "occupational problem" (V62.20) might apply.

5. The prognosis is good. The course of this disorder is generally time limited. Psychosocial stressors may disappear, resulting in rapid resolution of symptoms, or may continue, resulting in adaptation to a new level of functioning and a more gradual symptom resolution. If symptoms do not remit when the stressor ceases, another diagnosis should be considered.

PEARLS:

1. Adjustment disorders are common.

2. Axis IV of DSM-III is to specify what stressors are present and their severity.

3. Factors such as personality, culture, values and physical health influence one's response to stress and may increase vulnerability to adjustment disorders.

4. Stress, by definition, is a component of all adjustment disorders, though symptoms do not always begin immediately. By DSM-III criteria the symptoms must begin within three months.

PITFALLS:

1. The severity of the stress bears no relationship to the severity of one's emotional response. Very vulnerable individuals may react with extreme impairment to a mild stress, or conversely others may react mildly to an extreme stress.

2. The diagnosis of adjustment disorder does not apply to those with personality disorder whose symptoms get worse under stress (eg, the dependent individual who becomes more dependent after a divorce).

3. Uncomplicated bereavement is not considered an adjustment disorder. Impaired functioning is considered a normal reaction to the loss of a loved one.

4.   The busy practitioner will often prescribe minor tranquilizers for their adjustment disorder patients and
disregard the benefit of psychotherapy. Very few of
these patients are adequately treated by medication
alone.

TRIVIA:

Freud maintained that early childhood trauma (especially that occurring between ages 2 and 4) played a
major role in predisposing individuals to illness and
vulnerability to life stress.

REFERENCES

1.   American Psychiatric Association Task Force on Nomenclature and Statistics: Diagnostic and Statistical
Manual of Mental Disorders, 3rd ed. (DSM-III). Amer.
Psychiatric Association, Washington, DC, 1980.
2.   Axelrod J, Reisine TD: Stress hormones: Their inter-
action and regulation. Science 224:452-459, 1984.
3.   Goldberger L, Breznitz S: Handbook of Stress. New
York,   The Free Press, 1982.
4.   Horowitz MJ: Stress Response Syndromes. New York,
Jason Aronson, Inc., 1976.
5.   Kandel ER: From metapsychology to molecular biology:
Explorations into the nature of anxiety. Am J Psychiat
140:1277-1293, 1983.
6.   Kessler RC, Price RH, Wortman CB: Social factors in
psychopathology: Stress, social support, and coping
processes. Ann Rev Psychol 36:531-572, 1985.
7.   Robinson RG, Price TR: Post-stroke depressive disorders: A follow-up study of 103 outpatients. Stroke
13:635-641, 1982.

A PAIN IN THE NECK

CASE 34: A 36-year-old white, twice-married, construction
worker presents on referral from an orthopedic surgeon.
His chief complaint of upper back and neck pain dates back
three years to a time he fell from an 8-foot scaffolding.
The pain is described as dull, aching, non-radiating, worse
in the afternoons, better on weekends, benefited somewhat
by heat, intensified by lifting and anger, and entirely
absent some mornings. He has continued to work, but he
attempts to limit heavy lifting and has sharply curtailed
family activities with his wife and three children. Three
months ago he began using Percodan for "the real bad
times." Now he "requires" some at least daily.
      He denies all complaints except pain. However, his
mood seems depressed, affect is somber, and his outlook is
pessimistic. The surgeon's X-ray showed mild degenerative
and compression changes likely secondary to the trauma, yet
the pain seems out of proportion to the findings. That and
the increasing narcotic use prompted the referral.

QUESTIONS:

1.   What are the usual physiologic responses to acute pain
      and how do they change if the pain becomes chronic?

2.   How often are chronic pain patients depressed and how
      often do depressed patients complain of pain?

3.   What factors and psychological characteristics have
      been linked to those with chronic psychogenic pain
      (the pain-prone patient)?

4.   What is the characteristic MMPI profile of the chronic
      pain patient?

5.   Define "alexithymia." How does this concept relate to
      the chronic pain patient?

6.   What treatment is recommended for chronic pain
      patients?

ANSWERS:

1.   Physiologic responses to acute pain are identical to those of acute anxiety, i.e., increased respirations, increased blood pressure, increased heart rate, increased muscle tension, pupillary dilatation, and increased peripheral blood flow. If the pain continues, these responses often diminish and are replaced by depressive symptoms such as insomnia, anorexia, decreased energy, decreased sexual drive, and irritability.

2.   There is a high rate of concurrence between chronic pain and depression. The symptom picture is often similar and at times it is difficult to determine which is primary and which secondary. In one study (Lindsay, 1981) 87% of 300 chronic pain patients were also depressed and 57% of 196 patients in treatment for depression also complained of recurring pain.

3.   The experience of chronic pain may produce some of the psychological and emotional characteristics often seen in these patients, however, many experts favor the concept of the "pain-prone patient." This concept holds that chronic pain patients often demonstrate common psychological and life history features.
      The pain-prone patient often has an early history which includes physical abuse, aggressive alcoholic parent(s), parental attention limited to times of illness or suffering, and pain or illness in a parent. Onset of pain is often in adolescence where complaints of dysmenorrhea or a history of appendectomy without adequate justification are common. Life histories are often replete with failures and some contend that such patients have unconscious needs to continue the childhood pattern of defeat, hurt, and punishment. A curious finding in support of this notion is the observation of pain onset at times of apparent happiness and stability - as if the patient is not meant to experience contentment and pleasure. Psychodynamic theorists have postulated that some "pain-prone" patients are using pain as unconscious punishment for their guilt, while others unconsciously use it as a mechanism to bond them more closely to others. These mechanisms may derive from childhoods where guilt and punishment or punishment followed by over-affection were common themes. Common psychological features are pessimism, depression, guilt, dependency, and alexithymia (see question #5).

4. The characteristic MMPI profile shows elevations on clinical scales 1 (hypochondriasis), 2 (depression), and 3 (hysteria).

5. "Alexithymia" literally means "no words for feelings (or mood)" and refers to a person's inability to verbally communicate emotions and feelings. This trait has been linked to both somatizing and pain-prone patients, and in addition it implies emotional over-control, low psychological mindedness, stoicism, and limited creative mental fantasy. Some believe that patients with impaired ability to verbally and emotionally express their feelings are more likely to perceive and express them as aches, pains, and body dysfunctions.

6. Treatment of chronic pain should emphasize rehabilitation and restoration of function instead of complete cure. Treatment strategies are diverse and many modalities are commonly used in concert. Medications can be helpful. The tricyclic antidepressants have some specific analgesic properties (independent of their antidepressant properties) and are often beneficial at less than the usual antidepressant dosages. Neuroleptics have been recommended for the treatment of chronic pain, but this should be undertaken with caution since treatment is often lengthy - the possibility of tardive dyskinesia should be considered. A large percentage of chronic pain patients become addicted to narcotics and thus these medications should be used sparingly in the treatment of such pain. (However, in the treatment of the chronic pain of malignancy, narcotics are indicated and often underutilized.) Some patients are helped by transcutaneous nerve stimulation, acupuncture, nerve blocks, neurosurgery, and/or biofeedback, though most do not achieve permanent relief from these techniques. Behavior modification techniques may benefit chronic pain by increasing social activities, increasing physical activity and exercise, decreasing the use of analgesics, and modifying dependent behaviors and secondary gain. Traditional individual psychotherapy is generally ineffective except in those with a well-defined conflict as a significant etiologic factor. Group therapy is more effective, possibly through enhancing social activity, increasing interpersonal support, and encouraging self-reliance. Marriage and family therapy may be necessary to alter destructive family patterns and reinforcements.

The multidisciplinary pain clinic is one way of providing a comprehensive approach that has a high degree of acceptability among patients. Appropriate goals for such clinics appear to be (1) restoration of function, (2) decreased use of pain medications, (3) decreased use of medical care, (4) aiding the patient to understand and adapt to his situation, and (5) decreasing the patient's pain.

PEARLS:

1. A study of over 40,000 volunteers determined that (1) males tolerate considerably greater pain than females, (2) whites tolerate more pain than blacks who tolerate more pain than Orientals, (3) pain tolerance decreases with age for all races and both sexes.

2. Phantom pains and sensations occur in virtually 100% of limb amputees and follow about 50% of mastectomies. Persistent phantom pain appears to be strongly correlated with depression.

3. One of the most frequent complaints in the general population (18%) is back pain.

4. Pain is the most frequent presenting complaint to a physician.

5. Anxiety increases pain perception.

PITFALLS:

1. Pain is primarily subjective and defies all attempts at measurement or quantification.

2. Patients with psychogenic pain should not be treated as if their pain is not "real." Pain occurring for emotional reasons is not less real or painful.

3. The diagnosis of chronic pain does not always mean that some other emotional or personality disorder is present.

4. Most chronic pain patients have seen numerous physicians without benefit. Common errors are the assumption that previous physicians were simply incompetent. Don't adopt the patient's perspective that the pain represents some undiscovered somatic dysfunction.

5.   Not all chronic pain patients want to get better. Some desire doctor visits and repeated unsuccessful treatments as a means of blaming and manipulating others.

TRIVIA:

Solomon and Schmidt (1978) describe an interesting case of an amputee who experienced "burning" phantom limb pain after learning that (against his wishes) his severed limb had been disposed of by cremation.

REFERENCES

1.   Blumer D, Heilbronn M: The pain-prone disorder: A clinical and psychological profile. Psychosomat 22:395-402, 1981.
2.   Ford CV: The Somatizing Disorders: Illness as a Way of Life. New York, Elsevier Biomedical, 1983.
3.   Hendler N, et al: Group therapy with chronic pain patients. Psychosomat 22:333-340, 1981.
4.   Lindsay PG, Wyckoff M: The depression-pain syndrome and its response to antidepressants. Psychosomat 22: 571-577, 1981.
5.   Reich J, et al: Prediction of response to treatment in chronic pain patients. J Clin Psychiat 46:425-427, 1985.
6.   Reuler JB, Girard DE, Nardone DA: The chronic pain syndrome: Misconceptions and management. Ann Int Med 93:588-596, 1980.
7.   Solomon GF, Schmidt KM: A burning issue: Phantom limb pain and psychological preparation of the patient for amputation. Arch Surg 113:185-196, 1978.

"FASCINOMA"

<u>CASE 35</u>: You are called to consult on a 32-year-old white,
single male admitted to the hospital four weeks ago with
fever, hematuria and unusual bullous eruptions on the left
arm and thigh. The symptoms initially seemed to clear with
steroid therapy but they have now returned even more
intensely and the bullous eruption has spread to the left
chest.
    "He's been puzzling and fascinating," commented the
medicine intern. "Princess Diana of England is a distant
relative and he was being trained as a legal aide to the
British Parliament when he first got sick. That was five
years ago. Now he travels in this country as a curator for
a museum in Australia. His case is a real fascinoma. At
first we thought it was some atypical form of lupus but
that's been ruled out. The fever is really erratic and the
hematuria went away once on steroids, but now it's worse
than ever. His IVP is normal. The skin lesions are unlike
anything ever seen around here before. We're wanting a
psych consult because the pathologist says the skin
cultures are impossible. The first cultures showed a type
of Clostridia that he said was very unusual as a human
pathogen. Now he's growing out Lactobacillus and says it's
impossible."
    You examine the patient and find him to be pleasant
and cooperative. He talks freely with an engaging warmth
and no apparent thought or mood disorder. You leave him
after an hour without evidence of any specific psychiatric
disorder. As you sit at the nurses' station, one of the
nurses asks, "Did you see what he did when you left? When
I went in to take his temperature he pretended like he was
blowing a cavalry call on a trumpet and laughed, 'Send in
the shrinks, send in the shrinks. I was going to be a
shrink once but I got better.'"

COCKTAIL CLUE:

    At a cocktail party that evening you mention your
strange consultation to several doctors. One comments,
"Sounds like the guy we had at Memorial about a month
ago, only then he'd been a valet to Prince Charles and
was a scout for a New Zealand soccer team. We found
out he was shooting stuff under his skin and putting
blood in his urine samples."

QUESTIONS:

1. Should you search his room, attempt to secretly observe him, or do other things to try to prove deception?

2. What type of illness is this?

3. Should you confront the patient with your knowledge of what he is doing?

4. Should relatives, insurance companies, neighboring hospitals, and/or other physicians be alerted to this patient?

5. What is the prognosis?

ANSWERS:

1.   Generally <u>yes</u>, although such an approach has legal im-
        plications. Proper treatment will never be begun if
        the self-induced nature of the symptoms goes undis-
        covered. In this case it was arranged that the pa-
        tient would be taken to the laboratory the next morning
        for a urine sample obtained by catheterization. The
        specimen showed no hematuria or other abnormality.
        While he was away the hospital room was searched,
        yielding a needle, syringe and several finger lancets
        taped to the underside of the bed. Though never
        proven, it was strongly suspected that initially he
        had produced the unusual skin lesions by subdermally
        injecting a solution containing dirt from a plant in
        the room (which he had brought with him). Later, he
        likely injected milk, producing similar lesions but
        culturing out Lactobacillus rather than Clostridia.
        These lesions were probably confined to the left arm
        and chest because he was right-handed. The blood
        detected in the urine was probably obtained by finger
        lancet and added to each sample. Also, by description
        he was the same person who was at Memorial Hospital
        the previous month with similar symptoms.

2.   The patient's illness is <u>factitious</u>. "Factitious"
        means "produced artificially" and implies that sham
        symptoms (either physical or psychological) are delib-
        erately produced by the patient. Factitious illness
        is similar to <u>malingering</u> in that both involve the
        voluntary production of symptoms, but differs in that
        malingering involves a goal that is recognizable and
        motivated by some personal gain such as obtaining
        drugs or avoiding military duty. In factitious
        illness there is no apparent goal beyond adopting the
        patient role.
                Common characteristics of patients found to have
        factitious illness are: less than 40, unmarried, works
        or has worked in the medical field, psychological
        conflicts (commonly involving anger, sexuality,
        dependency or masochism), chaotic childhoods (often
        including disease or physical abuse), and personality
        disorder (often borderline personality). DSM-III
        divides factitious disorders into those with psycho-
        logical symptoms (Ganser syndrome) and those with
        physical symptoms. The most common factitious
        physical disorders are fever, dermatitides, blood
        disease (anemia and coagulation dyscrasias), endocrine
        disease (hyperthyroidism, hypoglycemia, and pheo-
        chromocytoma), and kidney stones.

An intense and extreme form of chronic factitious physical illness, likely shown by this patient, is the Munchausen syndrome where patients travel about seeking hospitalization, telling fantastic lies (pseudologia fantastica) and showing severe character pathology. The patient's cavalry call and "send in the shrinks" soliloquy is a clue to his personality disorder and suggests hostility, superiority and possibly feeling victorious in what he saw as a challenge with an adversary.

3. Yes. If any therapeutic relationship is to be established it must begin with an open discussion of what he is doing. Ideally, this discussion should precede the psychiatric consultation so as not to put the psychiatrist in a role as "the inquisitor" and impair his ability to form a therapeutic alliance. It is easy to feel angry and vindictive when deception is discovered, yet such an expression would be counterproductive. The most optimistic approach involves understanding that the patient is ill and in need of help, the expression that he must be distressed to seek medical care in such extreme ways, and the communication of a willingness to work with him.

   The patient's illness should not be denied, but rather redefined as psychological rather than physical. Even with an "ideal" approach, a positive response from the patient and good outcome in treatment is the exception rather than the rule.

4. This is a difficult ethical question which evades a simple non-controversial answer. The legal-ethical question is one of medical confidentiality and what are the rights of a patient who has perpetuated such fraud and deceit. Medical-legal opinion divides between two opposing views. One is that doctor-patient confidentiality cannot be unilaterally disregarded by the physician regardless of the circumstances and if the physical disagrees with the patient's conduct he should terminate his relationship. The other is that the patient's deceit, fraud, and abuse of trust negates the privileges that usually attend the doctor-patient relationship and strict "secrecy" only perpetuates the problem. A thoughtful evaluation of each situation should guide one's approach in this complex determination.

5. Poor. Such "illness behavior" is often a lifelong pattern that resists all treatment efforts. These patients commonly refuse psychiatric treatment and

seem to prefer this way of life despite its dangers
and uncertainties. When confronted with the opinion
of factitious illness they commonly become angry, deny
the possibility, threaten suits, and leave AMA to
continue the pattern elsewhere. In some patients,
acute single episode factitious illness seems related
to stress or underlying depression. Among these
patients the prognosis is much more optimistic.

PEARLS:

1. "The presence of factitious illness does not preclude
the coexistence of true psychological or physical
symptoms" (DSM-III, p 285).

2. According to one study the frequency of factitious
disorder is increasing. This may be related to the
higher proportion of medical care which is covered by
third party payers.

3. Factitious disease can occur in children but is uncommon.

4. Factitious disorder should be considered early in the
work-up of an adolescent with chronic unexplained
fever.

5. In 1979, 9% of patients referred to the National
Institutes of Health for fever of unknown origin
proved to have factitious fever.

6. "Munchausen by proxy" has been reported where mothers
repeatedly produce factitious illness in their children.

7. Factitious illness can simulate almost any physical
illness, limited only by the patient's intelligence
and medical knowledge.

8. Munchausen patients commonly travel between cities
seeking medical care. Some have been described
traveling between countries and continents.

9. Some patients use chronic benign physical or lab
findings (such as congenital nystagmus or an atypical
EEG) as objective support for their "illness."

PITFALLS:

1. The bizarre lifestyle and outlandish behavior of some
patients with factitious disorder leads to their being
misdiagnosed as schizophrenic.

2. Because fever is generally considered an objective indication of disease, its validity is not often questioned. In reality fever is one of the easiest symptoms to simulate or produce artificially.

3. Patients simulating illness will commonly allow (and often seek) dangerous diagnostic and treatment procedures even though they know the source of the symptom and the futility of the procedure.

4. Physicians often do not consider factitious illness in their differential diagnosis until a long and arduous work-up has excluded all other possibilities.

5. Reliable information on the causes of factitious illness is lacking, partly due to the reluctance of these patients to cooperate in evaluation, their tendency to run when discovered, and the questionable reliability of the histories given.

TRIVIA:

1. Baron Karl Friedrich Hieronymous von Munchausen was an 18th century German cavalry officer known for his extensive travels and entertaining and fantastic stories.

2. One well-studied 46-year-old Munchausen patient co-operated in obtaining his past medical records. They documented 400 hospitalizations. Another has been traced to 423 hospitalizations which included 102 upper GI series.

REFERENCES

1. Black D: The extended Munchausen syndrome: A family case. Brit J Psychiat 38:466-469, 1981.
2. Ford CV: The Somatizing Disorders: Illness as a Way of Life. New York, Elsevier Biomedical, 1983.
3. Ford CV, Abernathy B: Factitious illness: A multidisciplinary consideration of ethical issues. Gen Hosp Psychiat 3:329-336, 1981.
4. Pankratz L: A review of the Munchausen syndrome. Clin Psycholo Rev 1:65-78, 1981.
5. Rumans LW, Vosti KL: Factitious and fraudulent fever. Am J Med 65:745-755, 1978.
6. Shafer N, Shafer R: Factitious disease including Munchausen syndrome. NY State J Med 80:594-604, 1980.

CASE 36: A 26-year-old female, in town to visit relatives, is brought to the psychiatrist's office by a worried brother.

Over the preceding three days she has become exceptionally restless and now becomes agitated by almost any occurrence: the arrival of the mail at her brother's home causes her to shout and pound on the table about all the older people who receive no mail, and while shopping in the grocery store her sister-in-law finds her standing motionless, staring at the bread rack and muttering about how she must leave town and move to the country in order to help the farmers get a better price for their produce. She has been sleeping and eating little over the past week, and generally appears preoccupied.

More worrisome to the family, however, are the strange ideas she has developed. She is convinced that she has found the answer to "the AIDS mystery" and has filled two notebooks with scribblings about this topic during the last three days alone. She is convinced that gamma rays emanate from her fingertips and have healing powers, particularly if combined with her profound understanding of the motions of the planets.

The interview with the patient lasts less than five minutes. She can sit in a chair for only a few seconds. She jumps up, paces the room, picks up a pencil and writes something on a pad of paper, storms from the office, comes back, and leaves again - all in rapid-fire succession. Moreover, all this activity is accompanied by ceaseless, unintelligible mutterings, bursts of tears, and declarations of joy. She seems to understand the purpose of the interview but she also seems unable to control her emotions sufficiently to participate.

At this point, the brother adds some new information. Although neither the patient nor the family has a history of mental illness, six weeks earlier the patient had had a similar episode in her home town, was hospitalized for ten days, received a diagnosis of Bipolar Disorder, Manic (DSM-III 296.44), and was treated with thiothixene (Navane) and lithium. She got better quickly in the hospital but had unpleasant side effects from the Navane, so discontinued it after three weeks (although she continued to take the lithium faithfully), stopped therapy, and left town.

The patient was escorted directly from the office of the psychiatrist to a nearby hospital's psychiatric ward.

LABORATORY CLUE:

On the afternoon of admission, a stat blood lithium level was 1.2 meq/l. The next morning, the level was 0.5 meq/l, even though she had been placed on lithium 600 mg PO BID on admission.

QUESTIONS:

1. Was this woman with delusions and uncontrolled tearfulness really suffering from a manic episode?

2. Did she need hospitalization?

3. Why did her lithium level fall during the night following admission?

4. This was her second hospitalization in six weeks. What went wrong?

5. Name the two primary indications for lithium use.

6. What serum lithium level should you aim for in this patient?

7. On what lithium level should this patient be maintained?

ANSWERS:

1. Yes. The outstanding feature of her illness was an elevated, irritable mood that was accompanied by an increase in activity, flight of ideas, a decreased need for sleep, and distractibility. Grandiosity was present in her belief that she could "solve the AIDS mystery," her sense that she could cure with gamma rays, and her willingness to tackle the farm crisis single-handed.

    Delusional ideas (including paranoia), emotional lability (including crying), and bizarre behavior, far from being inconsistent with mania, are actually quite common in the fully developed state.

2. Yes. By the time she was brought for evaluation, she was almost incoherent and certainly couldn't function without her family's support. Even though she had been living with them for several weeks, her behavior was deteriorating rapidly (as is often the case in mania). Impulsive suicide during the nadir of an emotional swing or disastrous consequences stemming from exceptionally poor judgment (eg, believing they should be able to fly, they jump from a high window) make manic individuals potentially lethal if left unsupervised.

3. Although convinced that she had been taking her lithium faithfully, she had become so confused that she failed to recall the lithium she took just before reaching the psychiatrist's office. Thus, her lithium level was spuriously high (since lithium levels are based on blood drawn first thing in the morning, 12 hours after the evening dose). Her level the next morning (0.5 meq/l) confirmed a subtherapeutic level.

4. During her first hospitalization, she was placed on an antipsychotic (thiothixene) and lithium. Within ten days she had improved enough to be discharged. This improvement was most likely due to the Navane rather than to the lithium since lithium usually takes several weeks to become effective. Unfortunately, she stopped the Navane before she had stabilized on lithium, thus initiating the gradual deterioration.

5. Treatment of mania; Prophylaxis of bipolar AD. Lithium is the treatment of choice for manic individuals, although often an antipsychotic also must be used initially until the lithium becomes effective (as in this case). Lithium also prevents relapse of both the manic and depressive episodes of bipolar disorder.

There are a variety of other probable indications for lithium that are supported primarily by individual case reports: treatment of unipolar depression, cyclothymic disorder, and dysthymic disorder; prophylaxis of unipolar depression; treatment of selected patients with explosive disorder; etc. The specific indications for lithium are likely to increase in the future.

6. 1.0-1.2 meq/l. The risk of toxicity increases markedly above about 1.4 meq/l. On the other hand, effectiveness in controlling an acute episode is limited below about 0.9 meq/l.

7. 0.5-0.8 meq/l. The recommended maintenance level has been lowered in recent years as more patients have been found to be stable on doses in the 0.4-0.6 range.

PEARLS:

1. Bipolar illness has a lifetime risk of 1%, an equal sex distribution, an age of onset from the late teens through the early thirties, a <u>slight</u> tendency to occur in the upper classes and among the well educated, and clear evidence of genetic/biological roots.

2. Inter-individual differences in required oral dosage as well as in the pattern of toxic responses is great. Always individualize lithium treatment.

3. As a rule, younger patients require higher oral doses of lithium to maintain a therapeutic blood level.

4. The most common symptoms of lithium toxicity include lethargy and delirium progressing into stupor, neuromuscular irritability (hyperactive reflexes, fasciculations, myoclonic jerks), worsening tremor, and broken speech.

5. The effects on the kidney of long-term use of lithium have been exaggerated and usually shouldn't be a reason for discontinuing maintenance therapy. However, prolonged use does often result in a functional impairment in renal concentrating ability and occasionally a more long-lasting decline in the GFR. (In maintenance therapy, obtain a serum creatinine clearance and a 24-hour urine volume at least yearly.)

PITFALLS:

1. Some patients have mild side effects (most commonly a fine tremor and polyuria) even though their lithium

level is within the therapeutic range. Don't use the presence of those side effects as your dosing guide - rather, depend upon the blood level and clinical response.

2.   Pregnant women (particularly first trimester) should avoid lithium. Cardiac malformations are common in exposed infants. Moreover, lithium in the milk is 30-100% of maternal blood level.

TRIVIA:

During the 1940's lithium chloride was used by elderly individuals with heart failure as a replacement for table salt - until a number of deaths from lithium toxicity stopped the practice.

REFERENCES

1.   Climo LH: Treatment-resistant catatonic stupor and combined lithium-neuroleptic therapy: A case report. J Clin Psychopharmacology 5:166-170, 1985.
2.   Coryell W, Endicott J, Andreasen N, Keller M: Bipolar I, bipolar II, and nonbipolar major depression among the relatives of affectively ill probands. Am J Psychiatry 142:817-821, 1985.
3.   DePaulo JR: Lithium. In Clinical Psychopharmacology. Lake CR (Ed.), The Psychiatric Clinics of North Amer, Philadelphia, WB Saunders, September, 1984.
4.   Goodnick PJ, Fieve RR: Plasma lithium level and inter-episode functioning in bipolar disorder. Amer J Psychiatry 142:761-762, 1985.
5.   Lerer B: Alternative therapies for bipolar disorder. J Clin Psychiatry 46:309-316, 1985.

CASE 37: Ms. L, 35 years old and childless, lived alone and worked as a salesclerk after her recent divorce. She was unhappy and lonely. Moreover, she experienced a return of previous stomach pains which would often occur during pressured and demanding periods at work. In early December, as Christmas shopping increased her workload, she twice left her register complaining of pain and nausea. The manager referred her to a physician but seemed irritated and implied that if this problem continued, she should look for other employment.

She was displeased with her first appointment with the doctor. He was over an hour late, seemed rushed and uncaring, and after a cursory exam prescribed Tagamet for the pain. The medication helped initially, but as time went on the pain seemed unchanged. Her energy dropped. She began to lose weight and couldn't sleep. On follow-up, the physician seemed mildly annoyed that she was not improved. He focused on her insomnia complaint and prescribed Seconal, 100 mg at bedtime. The medication did help her sleep, but left her "hung over" in the morning and feeling even more depressed. Problems at work continued. Customers complained of her mistakes and inefficiency. She was fired from the job one afternoon and three days later was found dead in her apartment from a barbiturate overdose.

QUESTIONS:

1. What mental disorders predominate in those completing suicide?

2. Are persons who complete suicide usually under the care of a physician?

3. What personal and demographic factors are associated with increased suicide risk?

4. Are those who attempt suicide usually only crying for attention and do they rarely die by suicide?

ANSWERS:

1.   Diagnosis is a key risk factor in suicide assessment. Successful suicides show the following prevalence: depressive illness (50%), alcoholism (20%), schizophrenia (12%), and personality disorders (9%). Thus, about half of those who complete suicide are suffering from a potentially reversible condition - depression. Recent studies have also indicated that panic disorder imparts an increased suicide risk.

2.   Yes. Most people completing suicide have recently seen their physicians. A recent study found that 82% had seen their physicians within six months of their death and 53% within one month. Many of those who died by barbiturate overdose used medication recently prescribed by their physicians. Also, about two thirds had communicated their suicidal intentions to family, friends, or physicians - often in a clear and specific statement of their intent to die.

3.   Diagnosis (see question #1), living alone, poor health, chronic pain, unemployment, retirement, older age (over 45), white, male, and separated, widowed or divorced. In those younger than 45, high IQ may correlate with suicide risk. Also, important life stresses include recent change in dwelling, recent separation or divorce, and recent death of a loved one. Hopelessness and negative/pessimistic outlook toward the future also correlate with completed suicide.

4.   No. Persons who have attempted suicide are more likely than the general population to complete it at some later date. However, most who attempt suicide do not eventually die by suicide. The more serious the suicide attempt, the greater the correlation with eventual completed suicide.
      Of suicide attempters 2% kill themselves within a year and 10% eventually die by suicide (50-100 times that of the general population). The "usual" attempter is female, under 30, and without specific psychiatric diagnosis. The attempt is commonly impulsive, is relatively public, and uses a method which is of low lethality. Males complete suicide three times as often as females, while females attempt three times as often as males.

PEARLS:

1.   Of affective disordered patients 15% kill themselves.

2.   All of the major "functional" psychoses carry a significant risk of death by suicide (10-15%).

3.   Levels of CSF 5-hydroxyindoleacetic acid (5-HIAA - a serotonin metabolite) may prove to be a biologic marker for suicide. Studies have reported decreased levels in both depressed and non-depressed suicide attempters. A one-year follow-up showed 20% mortality by suicide in the "low 5-HIAA" group.

4.   Recent studies have supported the concept that genetic factors (independent of those associated with mental illness such as depression, alcoholism, and schizophrenia) play a role in the transmission of suicide behaviors. Exactly what the role is and how it operates is as yet unclear.

5.   Suicide rates are rising in the U.S. - particularly among the young (ages 15-29).

6.   Every person who attempts suicide should be seriously evaluated and most should be referred for treatment.

7.   Suicide is the 9th leading cause of death in the U.S. (11 certified suicides/100,000 population, but the actual number far exceeds this figure).

8.   Methods most commonly used in completed suicides are firearms, hanging, jumping, and drowning.

PITFALLS:

1.   Low danger to life in a first suicide attempt does not reliably predict low suicide risk in the future.

2.   Inquiring about suicide does not plant the idea or encourage suicide and, in fact, not to do so is a potentially dangerous attitude for a physician.

3.   Many physicians treat potential depressive complaints such as insomnia, fatigue, or pain without inquiring deeply enough to make a diagnosis of depression. Such treatment is incorrect.

4.   Passage of a crisis or beginning improvement of depressive symptoms does not indicate that the suicide danger is over. It is sometimes at this point that one has the energy and determination to make the attempt.

REFERENCES

1. Clayton PJ: Epidemiologic and risk factors in suicide. In Grinspoon L (Ed.), <u>Psychiatry Update</u>, Washington, DC, American Psychiatric Press, 1983.
2. Coryell W, Noyes R, Clancy J: Excess mortality in panic disorder. Arch Gen Psychiat 39:701-703, 1982.
3. Resnick HPL: Suicide. In Kaplan HI, Freedman AM, Sadock BJ (Eds.), <u>Comprehensive Textbook of Psychiatry III</u>, Baltimore, Williams & Wilkins, 2085-2098, 1980.
4. Roy A: Family history of suicide in affective disorder patients. J Clin Psychiat 46:317-319, 1985.
5. Traskman L, et al: Monoamine metabolites in CSF and suicidal behavior. Arch Gen Psychiat 38:631-636, 1981.

CASE 38: A 56-year-old man was admitted to the hospital with a diagnosis of major depression. Over the previous 4 months he had been treated as an outpatient at a rural community mental health center. He had originally presented there with irritability, anxiety, and mild depression and had been treated with weekly psychotherapy and three 6-week trials of antidepressants (including an MAO inhibitor).

His condition worsened. He became increasingly withdrawn, voiced suicidal ideas, began to move slowly (psychomotor retardation was identified by his therapist), and, by the time of his admission, was almost mute.

On admission, he appeared profoundly depressed and modestly confused. He replied slowly and incompletely to questions. He was oriented X 3 but showed confused judgment and impaired recent memory.

Sensing a medical problem, all medications were stopped and laboratory studies were initiated. Routine labs (CBC with differential, UA, VDRL, chest X-ray) were normal as was a cerebral CT scan. An EEG showed diffuse slowing. T_3, T_4, vitamin B_{12}, and folate levels were normal. A careful physical exam was unremarkable except for slight ataxia, fine tremors of the fingers of both hands, irregular pupils with sluggish reflexes, and hyperactive tendon reflexes.

QUESTIONS:

1. What should you do now?

2. What is the likely diagnosis?

3. How do you explain the negative VDRL?

4. What is the pathological picture?

5. How would you treat this patient?

ANSWERS:

1.   An LP. Clearly there is something wrong with cerebral function that is slowly progressive and that isn't evident in CNS anatomy (ie, the CT scan).
     The LP results were:
         glucose - nl
         protein - 85 mg%
         cells   - 40/mm^3 (mostly lymphocytes)
         VDRL   - negative
         FTA-ABS - positive

2.   Paretic neurosyphilis (general paresis). This is the "great mimic" of psychiatric conditions; the form of tertiary neurosyphilis most likely to present with emotional symptoms (although both meningeal syphilis and meningovascular syphilis can produce behavioral symptomatology).
     The diagnosis depends upon positive CSF serology, increased cells and protein in the CSF, and psychiatric symptoms which can range from dementia (most common) to depression (next most common), mania, anxiety, personality changes, psychosis, impotence, conversion symptoms, etc. Neurological signs and symptoms are often present as well, particularly pupillary changes such as the Argyll-Robertson pupil (small, irregular, nonreactive to light but constricts on accommodation and convergence).

3.   Reagin tests for syphilis, such as the VDRL, are negative in about 30% of patients with neurosyphilis. Moreover, false positives may be produced by a variety of conditions including drug abuse, acute infections, collagen diseases, malaria, hepatitis, and old age. More reliable (but also more time-consuming and costly) are the treponemal serologic tests like the FTA-ABS. They should be used for confirmation if neurosyphilis is suspected, whether or not the VDRL is positive.

4.   Menigneal thickening with accompanying parenchymal involvement of the brain, neuronal loss, and cerebral atrophy. The frontal and temporal lobes are affected preferentially (as might be suspected from the psychiatric symptoms).

5.   Untreated, most neurosyphilis patients die within four years. Treated successfully, symptom progression stops in almost all cases and significant improvement occurs in about 40% (dementia is least likely to reverse).

Penicillin is the drug of choice. It was once thought that a several-day course of high dose (several million units) IM antibiotics was sufficient; however, we now know that this does not sterilize the CSF in all cases. Current recommendations are for up to 24 million units of crystalline penicillin G daily, IV, for two weeks.

PEARLS:

1. In one study, 300 mental health center outpatients were screened for neurosyphilis and five previously unsuspected cases were found, all in patients between the ages of 50-60.

2. At the turn of the century, 10% of patients in mental hospitals had general paresis; today, it is unusual.

3. Syphilis is on the rise, particularly among the homosexual population. Thus, we may encounter more tertiary forms in the next several decades. However, because of the frequent use of low doses of antibiotics for a variety of minor medical conditions, the clinical picture of paretic neurosyphilis may be changing in unpredictable ways.

4. Perhaps as many as one third of patients with CNS syphilitic infection are asymptomatic.

5. General paresis teaches us that a careful physical exam is always required on seriously ill psychiatric patients.

PITFALLS:

1. Do not forget about general paresis just because its incidence has declined dramatically in recent decades. It is still around.

2. A slight contamination of an LP sample with the patient's FTA-ABS positive blood will produce a false positive test on the CSF, giving the incorrect impression that neurosyphilis is present.

TRIVIA:

The writers Baudelaire and de Maupassant, the composers Schubert and Schumann, the artist Gauguin, the philosopher Nietzsche, and the politician Lord Randolph Churchill (Winston Churchill's father) all died of neurosyphilis.

REFERENCES

1. Adams RD, Victor M: Principles of Neurology. New York, McGraw-Hill, 1985.
2. Dijkstra JWE: Asymptomatic neurosyphilis. Intern J Derm 22:581-589, 1983.
3. Gimenez-Roldan S: Neurosyphilis - Old and new problems. Hexagon (Roche) 13 (1):8-14, 1985.
4. Gomez EA, Aviles M: Neurosyphilis in community mental health clinics: A case series. J Clin Psychiat 45:127-129, 1984.
5. Lee JB, Kim SC, et al: Symptomatic neurosyphilis. Intern J Derm 22:577-580, 1983.
6. Lishman WA: Organic Psychiatry. Oxford, Blackwell, 1978.
7. Rundell JR, Wise MG: Neurosyphilis: A psychiatric perspective. Psychosomatics 26:287-295, 1985.

<u>CASE 39</u>:   Mr. Samuels, a 71-year-old, white, married, retired city health inspector is brought for an outpatient evaluation by his 70-year-old wife. The patient says he doesn't know why he is here. His wife says she wants "one more checkup before we put him in the nursing home."

The patient had been in good health until about three months ago.   By his wife's report he had been a hard worker, a good husband and father, and, except for a few episodes of mild depression, had seemed happy and well adjusted. He retired from his city job at age 65 and began what seemed to be an enjoyable retirement. He loved gardening and attended the spa and local library daily.   At age 70, he volunteered to go to Texas with his wife as a religious missionary. Not very interested in going, he did so to please his wife. His first two months of preaching seemed to go well. Then, three months ago, he complained of not feeling well and said he could no longer remember the lessons that he was supposed to teach. He began to refuse to keep his appointments saying, "My mind goes blank. I'm losing my memory. I can't remember anymore." Next, he began getting disoriented in his own apartment and often was unable to find the bathroom or kitchen.   After two weeks of this, he was taken to a local general practice physician. His memory was found to be impaired, he could not perform serial sevens, his fund of information was poor, and he was disoriented to time and place. The doctor diagnosed "Dementia - probably Alzheimer's disease," and recommended that they terminate their religious mission, return home, and begin making preparations to have Mr. Samuels placed in a nursing home.   Now that they have returned home, Mrs Samuels wants a psychiatrist to see him and wishes some help in arranging for the nursing home.

MENTAL STATUS CLUES:

>Presentation: Rather carelessly dressed and groomed
>with solemn affect and complaints of poor memory
>and concentration.
>
>Orientation: Disoriented to date (one month off). He
>knows the city he is in but not the building or
>address. Well oriented to person.
>
>Memory: Recent and remote memory appear equally
>impaired.
>
>Attention: No obvious impairment.
>
>Serial Sevens: "93, 87, I don't know. I can't do
>numbers anymore."
>
>Presidents: "I don't know. My memory is gone."
>
>Calculations: "4 + 3 = 7, 4 X 3 = I don't know, 6 + 7
>= 13, 6 X 7 = 47, 8 X 9 = I can't do it, 8 X 12 =
>96, 12/3 = I don't know."

QUESTIONS:

1.   What type of dementia does this patient have?

2.   What points from the history are consistent with the diagnosis?

3.   Does the mental status exam support this diagnosis?

4.   What would prove beyond reasonable doubt that this is the correct diagnosis?

5.   What is the prognosis in this disorder?

ANSWERS:

1. The patient has <u>pseudodementia</u>, which, of course, is not a dementia at all. This is a syndrome in which patients with other psychiatric disorders (most often depression) have symptoms which mimic true dementia. Mistaking a depression for dementia is always detrimental to the patient. The depression, a highly treatable condition, goes untreated; the prognosis is assumed to be poor and so little diagnostic or therapeutic effort is expended; and the patient may be placed in a custodial facility where the dreary and unstimulating environment weighs even further against recovery.

   The depressed elderly often don't complain overtly of depressive symptoms such as sadness, crying, guilt, or wanting to die. As in this case, a "dementia-like" picture of poor memory, loss of initiative, confusion, disorientation, and loss of interest, irritability, or concentration can predominate. The cognitive dysfunction associated with severe depressive illness can be indistinguishable from diffuse organic disease.

2. Historical points suggesting pseudodementia are: short duration of symptoms; rapid onset of symptoms; past history of depression; much complaining from the patient about cognitive dysfunction; and his highlighting failures, not trying to keep up, and emphasizing disabilities.

3. Yes. Mental status findings which suggest pseudodementia are: equal impairment of recent and remote memory, frequent "I don't know" responses, not trying on many items, variable performance (such as his missing or not trying on simple math problems while responding correctly to more difficult ones), and relative preservation of attention.

4. Consistent historical and mental status findings are suggestive as is an abnormal dexamethasone suppression test (DST), however, the diagnosis should be considered proven only when the underlying psychiatric cause has been reversed and the cognitive symptoms have resolved.

5. The prognosis is good if the correct diagnosis is made. Successful treatment of the underlying psychopathology often reverses the cognitive dysfunction. Mr. Samuels was treated with ECT and responded completely.

If the dementia is taken at face value, the outlook is much less favorable. Institutionalizing such patients may lead to increased intellectual impairment, further mental decline, physical deterioration, and even death.

PEARLS:

1. The incidence of severe depression in the elderly is estimated to be about 15%.

2. In the United States, the elderly comprise about 11% of the population and about 25% of suicides.

3. About 25% of "true dementia" patients are also depressed, and pseudodementia superimposed on true dementia has been reported as well.

4. "I don't know," "I don't remember," and "I can't do it" are answers characteristic of pseudodementia.

5. A past history of affective episodes should increase one's suspicion that dementia-like symptoms are secondary to a depression.

6. Rapid onset, short duration of symptoms, vociferous complaints, and self-reproach favor pseudodementia.

7. Dementia-like presentations in the elderly may be secondary to medication.

PITFALLS:

1. On follow-up, 10-20% of the elderly who were diagnosed as having mild dementia actually had depression.

2. If an initial depressive episode goes untreated, subsequent episodes often become progressively more severe.

3. Depressive symptoms in the elderly can be dismissed by the uninformed or prejudiced as "just a normal part of growing old."

TRIVIA:

The first description of a pseudodementia was by Ganser in 1898.   He described prisoners who seemed demented but weren't.   He felt the cause was either malingering or hysterical behavior and observed that the symptoms resolved when their legal problems ended (Ganser's syndrome).

REFERENCES

1.   Chaisson-Stewart GM: <u>Depression in the Elderly</u>. New York, John Wiley & Sons, 1985.
2.   Janowsky DS: Pseudodementia in the elderly: differential diagnosis and treatment. J Clin Psychiatry 43:9, 1982.
3.   McAllister TW: Overview: Pseudodementia. Am J Psychiatry 140:528-533, 1983.
4.   Wells CE: Pseudodementia and recognition of organicity. In Benson DF, Fullmer D (Eds.), <u>Psychiatric Aspects of Neurological Disease, Vol II</u>. New York, Grune & Stratton, 167-178, 1982.
5.   Wells CE, Duncan GW: <u>Neurology for Psychiatrists</u>. Philadelphia, FA Davis Co, 1980.

CASE 40:   Dr. Levin, a medicine resident, requested
psychiatric consultation and treatment for Mrs. R, an
inpatient with end-stage kidney failure. She is 45 years
old, divorced, and has chronic, bilateral pyelonephritis
which has progressed to virtual non-function. She has had
six months of renal dialysis and apparently had adjusted
well to the rigors and restrictions of her three-times-a-
week treatments, although she has seemed a little
demoralized since her medical leave from work was converted
to a medical retirement two weeks ago.

Her current admission to the nephrology service
resulted when her 17-year-old son found her in a semi-
comatose state. In the emergency room she had profound
hyperkalemia (8.5 meq/l) and was admitted for immediate
dialysis. Now, two days later, her medical condition is
stable. She was scheduled to be discharged today, but
seemed depressed on morning rounds and psychiatry was asked
to consult before she leaves the hospital.

Psychiatric examination is consistent with a depression of approximately six months duration. She presents
with depressed facies, slow speech, agitated handwringing,
and teary eyes. Complaints include insomnia, anorexia,
fatigue, and low sexual interest that are worse than the
"usual" amount of these symptoms which accompanied her
renal disease. She talks of a profound apathy, daily
crying spells, guilt, worthlessness, and hopelessness, all
of which are unlike her prior jovial nature. At this point
in the interview she bursts into tears and cries, "I've
even wanted to die. I can't go on like this." There is no
evidence of psychotic thinking or cognitive impairment.
Past history is negative for previous depressive episodes.
Family history includes an alcoholic father, an uncle who
committed suicide, and a sister who takes "some kind of
medicine for bad depressions."

CLUE:

Dangerous hyperkalemia is an uncommon event in the
well-managed dialysis patient.

QUESTIONS:

1.   Should this woman be cleared for discharge?

2.   What psychological stresses are associated with renal
      failure and dialysis?

3.   What psychiatric complications are associated with
      renal failure and dialysis?

4.   Should this patient, or any other in renal failure, be
      treated with antidepressant medication?

5.   What was the cause of her high serum potassium on
      admission?

ANSWERS:

1. No. Her depression is obviously severe and requires treatment. She is probably unable to manage on her own. In addition, since she is divorced and her son is often away at school, she lacks support and monitoring. Suicide in a severely depressed, divorced, unemployed, chronically ill person is a major risk.

2. Despair and uncertainty accompany any serious chronic illness. However, renal failure/dialysis patients have the additional burden of being bound to a machine until successful transplant or death. This is especially difficult for a patient who had previously been ambitious and independent. Such forced dependency on medical personnel and a time-consuming procedure (10-20 hours/week) often leads to frustration, resistance, anger, depression, and anxiety. Moreover, many dialysis patients find it stressful to see their blood leave their body, go through a machine, and return. (Mrs. R had commented, "that's something I'll never get used to.") Finally, most dialysis patients know that medical complications, including strokes and seizures, may occur during a dialysis run.

    The dialysis patient's life centers around these life-sustaining daily routines. They can never fully forget that they are seriously ill. When not on dialysis they must carefully adhere to medication and dietary requirements (low salt, low protein, low potassium, and low fluid). Loss of jobs (2/3 do not return to full-time work), personal freedom, income, self-esteem, financial security, sexual pleasure, and years of life expectancy all take an emotional toll. In addition, many dialysis patients never feel fully well because of mild degrees of uremia, anemia, electrolyte imbalance, or other medical complications. Since these stresses involve the spouse and family as well, they often lead to marriage and family turmoil.

3. Depression is the most common psychiatric complication. This often goes untreated, both due to physicians'lack of knowledge as well as the opinion that such depressed feelings are to be expected. Both attempted and completed suicide are more common among dialysis patients. Many experience anxiety in response to life changes, stresses, uncertainties, and the dialysis procedure itself. Sexual difficulties are present in most dialysis patients and are likely related to both organic and psychological factors. Family discord, with depression and anxiety in family members, is also common. Psychosis occurs infrequently.

4.   Yes. This patient presents a host of findings that
      predict benefit from antidepressant medication
      (disturbances of sleep, appetite, libido, and energy;
      agitation; and family history of depressive disorders).
      A common impediment to proper treatment is the incor-
      rect assumption by many physicians that antidepressant
      medications are contraindicated in patients with renal
      failure. Many patients with renal disease who would
      benefit from psychotropic medication never receive it.
          Tricyclic antidepressants are largely metabolized
      by the liver and are not removed from the blood by
      dialysis. They can and should be used in appropriate
      renal failure patients. Dosage should be initiated
      and increased cautiously and be monitored by periodic
      blood levels. The appropriate dose is usually about
      2/3's that given to a patient with normal kidney
      function.

5.   Mrs. R had attempted suicide by a "potassium binge"
      and by missing dialysis. After transfer to the
      psychiatry service she confessed during group therapy
      that she had "overdosed" on bananas and grape juice
      and had missed two dialysis sessions after telling her
      regular dialysis personnel that she would be away for
      a few days and would be dialyzed at another center.
      This is not an uncommon method of suicide in the
      dialysis patient. In a large study of suicide and
      dialysis (3,500 patients), 17 committed suicide by
      active means, 17 attempted suicide, and 117 died from
      failure to adhere to their medical regimen.

PEARLS:

1.   Patients with well functioning kidney transplants need
      no special consideration regarding psychotropic use
      except for additional caution regarding any nephrotox-
      icity.

2.   About 3,500 Americans develop renal failure yearly (15
      per 100,000 per year).

3.   The number of patients treated by dialysis or trans-
      plant is increasing rapidly. The 25,000 such patients
      in 1983 represent a 23% increase over 1980.

4.   Of men on dialysis, 70% are sexually impotent.

5.   Antipsychotics may be used in the dialysis patient
      with cautious monitoring. The usual dosage is about
      2/3 that given when kidney function is normal.

6.   Lithium may be used in a dialysis patient despite its being both dialyzable and primarily excreted by the kidneys. A dose of about 600 mg following each dialysis run is usually sufficient to produce an adequate blood level which remains until it is removed by the next dialysis.

PITFALLS:

1.   The recent idea that dialysis is a useful treatment for schizophrenia is incorrect - don't use it.

2.   In renal failure patients, avoid using benzodiazepines which have active metabolites (such as diazepam and chlordiazepoxide). Benzodiazepines with no active metabolites (such as lorazepam and oxazepam) may be used with care at about 2/3 the usual dosage.

3.   Failure to use appropriate psychotropic medication in the dialysis patient is a much more common problem than adverse or untoward effects from such medications

REFERENCES

1.   Abram HS, et al: Suicidal behavior in chronic dialysis patients. Amer J Psychiatry 127:1199-1214, 1971.
2.   Bennett WM, et al: Drug therapy in renal failure: Dosing guidelines for adults: Part II. Sedatives, hypnotics, and tranquilizers; cardiovascular, anti-hypertensive and diuretic agents; miscellaneous agents. Ann Intern Med 93:286-325, 1980.
3.   Levy NB: Use of psychotropics in patients with kidney failure. Psychosomatics 26:699-709, 1985.
4.   Levy NB: Psychological reactions to machine dependency: Hemodialysis. Psychiatr Clin North Am 4:351-363, 1981.
5.   Port FK, et al: Lithium therapy during maintenance hemodialysis. Psychosomatics 20:130-131, 1979.

CASE 41: A shy, socially awkward, painfully well-behaved 17-year-old male attended a high school graduation party. During the party he was teased unmercifully by his peers for being a prude. Midway through the evening he became enraged, began to shout incomprehensibly, and attacked several males and females who stood nearby. He was physically subdued and, still shouting, was wrestled into a car for a trip to the hospital.

In the emergency room, he thought he was in an airplane and fought with those nearby to keep from being hurled out the door to his death. When his parents arrived he recognized them but was too agitated to communicate in any meaningful way. He was suspicious and fearful of the ER staff and was hyperalert to surrounding activity. A determined physical and neurological exam (such as could be done) was unremarkable except for prominent diaphoresis and flushing. Because of the uncertainty about the diagnosis, no medication was prescribed. Rather, it was decided to put him in a low stimulation environment with close observation.

Although no history could be obtained from the patient (and the "friends" who had brought him to the ER had long since departed), his parents related that he had always been a model son who was a good student and had never had any emotional problems save for some mild depressions apparently related to his inability to maintain close friends. He had never been in trouble with the law and never used alcohol or drugs. Moreover, there was no family history of serious emotional illness.

In the hour it took to obtain the relevant history from his parents, the patient had gradually become less agitated and, in fact, was responding lethargically. He remained confused and the ER personnel were concerned that he was slipping into a stuporous state. The routine blood work and urinalysis obtained upon admission was normal and the urine drug screen was not back yet. He was sent for a "stat" EEG.

CLINICAL CLUE:

The EEG was read as "generalized slowing of delta waves with bursts of theta activity."

QUESTIONS:

1.   What caused this patient's sudden symptoms?

2.   What is the likely offending agent?

3.   Name 15 street terms for compounds containing this drug.

4.   How would you make the diagnosis?

5.   How would you treat this patient?

ANSWERS:

1. Probably an unsuspected drug ingestion. Other psych-
    iatric illnesses generally do not present this sudden-
    ly, without warning or obvious precipitants. Although
    a shy, controlled individual placed under stress could
    have reacted with an explosive outburst, it is unlike-
    ly that he would have become disoriented or that such
    rage and disorientation would have continued following
    his transfer to the emergency room.
        Other, less likely, possibilities include a toxic,
    delirious reaction to some foreign substance, a
    sudden medical or neurological illness, or a seizure
    phenomenon, although nothing suggesting any of these
    was uncovered during his evaluation in the ER.

2. <u>Phencyclidine</u> or PCP. (It was slipped into his coke
    for a joke.)

3. Angel dust, angel hair, Cadillac, CJ, crystal, dust,
    elephant tranquilizer, hog, embalming fluid, killer
    weed, peace pill, pocket fuel, super grass, zombie
    dust, devil dust.

4.   The diagnosis in this case, as in most PCP cases,
    depends upon four factors.

    <u>History</u> of drug ingestion - Although the patient was
    not aware that he had been given the drug, a later
    check with others at the party revealed that he had
    been slipped "some dust to loosen him up."

    <u>Symptoms</u> - Symptoms of PCP use are dose-related. Low
    doses produce a mixture of excitement, racing thoughts,
    anxiety/panic, paranoia, strange behaviors, and sen-
    sory changes such as numbness (PCP is, after all, an
    anesthetic), parasthesias, and illusions. Moderate
    doses produce lethargy, muscular rigidity, gross inco-
    ordination, generalized nystagmus, diaphoresis, fever,
    and hyperacousis. High doses can produce stupor,
    coma, and death. This patient obviously had received
    a significant dose since, after approximately 1 1/2
    hours, he was becoming stuporous.

    The <u>EEG</u> - Slowed delta and altered theta activity is
    common (but, unfortunately, not pathognomonic). There
    is seldom justification for doing an EEG "stat."

    Urine or gastric aspirate <u>PCP levels</u> - PCP is a weak
    base which becomes ionized <u>in an acid</u> medium and then
    trapped because the ion can't pass through biological

membranes. Thus, PCP becomes concentrated in the acid stomach and in the urine (particularly if the urine is acid).

5. Place in a low sensory environment (quiet, low level of lighting). Treat agitation with a major tranquilizer such as haloperidol or a benzodiazepine. Provide gastric lavage and continuous gastric drainage. Encourage elimination of PCP by acidifying the urine to a pH below 5.0 (oral cranberry juice and ascorbic acid).

PEARLS:

1. During the mid 1970's, PCP was the leading drug of abuse in the United States. Its use is currently declining.

2. PCP is a water-soluble, white powder which can be made easily and cheaply in a "basement laboratory."

3. PCP is currently available as the veterinary anesthetic and tranquilizer Sernylan.

4. PCP crosses the placental barrier and can produce a toxic syndrome in newborns which includes vomiting and diarrhea, jitteriness, and hypertonicity.

5. During the 1950's, many of the normal volunteers who received IV PCP as part of a large trial of the drug's effects developed a psychotic state which closely mimicked acute schizophrenia.

6. Complications from severe overdoses can include hypertension with hypertensive encephalopathy, respiratory arrest, myoglobinuria from rhabdomyolysis, and even renal failure. Occasional comatose patients have recovered after remaining on mechanical assistance for several days.

7. When ingested, the onset of action is in 15-30 minutes. When smoked, it is within 5 minutes. (The half-life of PCP is 30-60 minutes.)

8. Tolerance develops - the chronic PCP user requires increasing doses for the same effect - although withdrawal symptoms have not been noted.

9. Unlike the patient with an acute ingestion of PCP, the chronic user often has negligible amounts of PCP in the urine and gastric aspirate.

PITFALLS:

1. It is often difficult to differentiate a chronic PCP psychosis from schizophrenia reactivated by PCP. However, some experts argue that only those individuals who are predisposed to schizophrenia will develop a chronic psychosis with PCP use.)

2. Don't assume that a patient has recovered when he has been clear for 24 hours and has low or undetectable serum PCP levels - the patient with a serious overdose may need to remain in the hospital for several days to a week before you can be sure that he has recovered. (Moreover, the chronic PCP user may develop a delirious state lasting for several weeks.) Patients with PCP overdoses often follow a waxing and waning course over a period of days. This is probably due to both the high lipid solubility of PCP (thus it is concentrated in fatty tissues and the brain, with comparatively low levels in the serum) and gastroenteric recirculation (concentrated from the blood into the acid stomach and then reabsorbed in the alkaline intestine).

REFERENCES

1. Aronow R, Done AK: Phencyclidine overdose: An emerging concept of management. J Am Coll Emer Physicians 7:56-59, Feb., 1978.

2. Castellani S, Giannini AJ, Adams PM: Physostigmine and haloperidol treatment of acute phencyclidine intoxication. Am J Psychiatry 139:508-510, 1982.

3. Domino EF: PCP (Phencyclidine); Historical and Current Perspectives. Ann Arbor, MI, NPP Books, 1981.

4. Dove HW: Phencyclidine: Pharmacologic and clinical review. Psychiatric Medicine 2(2):189-209, 1984.

5. Nabeshima T, Yamaguchi K, et al: Serotonergic involvement in phencyclidine-induced behaviors. Pharm Biochem & Behav 21:401-408, 1984.

CASE 42: A 32-year-old man arrived 20 minutes late for his first psychiatric appointment, having gotten lost trying to find the office. His request for evaluation represented just one in a long series of attempts to get help: he had seen (by rough count) 13 psychiatrists and psychologists over the preceding 9 years and had undergone two courses of "intensive psychotherapy," each lasting longer than one year. He had received many diagnoses including dysthymic disorder, anxiety neurosis, explosive disorder, borderline personality, latent schizophrenia, "neurotic," and "seriously neurotic." He had been treated with extensive psychotherapy of several different types (primarily psychodynamic, client-centered, and behavioral) and had received trials of several medications (primarily benzodiazepines, tricyclics, and phenothiazines), all without significant benefit. His expectation for successful treatment was low and, as he unfolded his history of past treatments, so became that of his new psychiatrist.

By his report, he has had "just about every symptom in the book." He has been depressed off and on for as long as he can remember; moreover, another bout of depression is the reason for once again seeking help. He feels his depressions have resulted from his life "going nowhere." A bright, likable fellow, he has been fired from innumerable jobs and has been divorced three times. He has displayed a pattern of "sounding off" to authority and losing his temper which has cost him many desirable jobs. Moreover, his episodes of severe impatience and temper outbursts have formed the basis for each of his divorces. (Because of "rage-like" episodes, he has been evaluated neurologically for a seizure disorder, to no avail.) He admits to becoming frustrated and losing his temper easily but notes, disgustedly, "You would too if nothing ever went your way."

He also has suffered from frequent episodes of anxiety without panic attacks and has dealt with those episodes, unsuccessfully, by drinking too much (another criticism of his former wives). Much of his past psychotherapy has been directed at helping him understand why he feels and acts these ways. Although he believes that he has learned much about himself through this process, his behavior and his problems remain essentially unchanged.

His problems have been with him since childhood. As a grade school student he was unruly, fought frequently, and was often the subject of disciplinary action. He barely finished high school and, although tested to have an IQ "somewhere above 130," he couldn't settle down sufficiently to complete even one year of college. He had two arrests as a minor for "breaking and entering" but has had no dif-

ficulties since. Except for his episodic alcohol use, he
has not used alcohol or drugs to any extent. There is no
family history of emotional disorders although, according
to his mother, he is "just like his father" who died in an
industrial accident when the patient was 12.

The patient is currently asking for help. His mental
status examination is unremarkable. He is pleasant,
cooperative, and goal oriented. He is intelligent, his
memory is good, and he shows no signs of organicity. There
is no evidence of psychotic thinking. At the end of your
evaluation, he asks you if you have anything to offer him.

QUESTIONS:

1. Should you tell him to save his money - that the last
    thing he needs is more psychotherapy and more meds,
    since they both have been proven valueless to him?

2. What can you offer him?

3. How would you confirm such a diagnosis?

4. What medications are potentially useful?

ANSWERS:

1.   No. In fact, you have a perspective that may be of
      significant value to him - one which can be tested
      both quickly and inexpensively.

2.   A new diagnostic possibility: Attention Deficit Disor-
      der, Residual Type (ADD-R), DSM-III 314.80.

      The "hyperactive child syndrome" is now known as
      Attention Deficit Disorder with Hyperactivity or ADDH.
      ADD-R represents the acknowledgement that hyperactivi-
      ty in children does not disappear with adolescence as
      was formerly thought but can remain symptomatic well
      into adulthood (greater than 50% of children). Accord-
      ing to DSM-III, although hyperactivity per se disap-
      pears, a variety of symptoms persist from childhood
      including "difficulty organizing work and completing
      tasks, difficulty concentrating, being easily distrac-
      ted, and making sudden decisions without thought of
      the consequences."
      Additional research suggests that many of these
      "hyperactive children grown up" continue to be restless
      and irritable as well. They often have problems with
      continuing temper outbursts and impulsivity which
      causes problems in their marriages, their jobs, and
      with interpersonal relations in general. Moreover, a
      common theme with many of these patients is chronic
      dysphoria and a sense of low self-worth, perhaps due
      to life-long criticism of their behavior by others.

3.   This diagnosis requires a high index of suspicion
      since the characteristic behavior is so easily
      explained by other diagnoses (as was the case with
      this patient). These patients will often be thought
      to suffer from a primary mood disorder (either depres-
      sion or mania - and thus be treated with antidepres-
      sants or lithium), a neurotic problem (and thus be
      treated with psychotherapy and medications like benzo-
      diazepines), a primary anxiety disorder, or a pre-
      psychotic condition (and be treated with antipsycho-
      tics).
      There is no pathognomonic symptom, but a history
      of typical hyperactive behavior in childhood which has
      continued to the present and a family history of
      similar difficulties is very suggestive. Equally
      indicative of ADD-R is a positive medication trial.

4.   Stimulants (eg, methylphenidate) can produce rapid,
      remarkable improvements in certain ADD-R patients. In
      a matter of a day or two, many of their life-long

symptoms and behaviors may improve dramatically, thus
confirming the diagnosis. Such medication may then be
useful for long-term treatment. However, we are not
yet able to identify with certainty those ADD-R patients most likely to respond to stimulants.

A problem with the use of stimulants for treatment of this condition is that this class of medication is both abusable and valuable. Thus, individual
patients must be selected carefully for pharmacological
treatment since this group of impulsive, irritable,
labile patients are at risk for either addiction or to
sell the medication for profit.

PEARLS:

1. Of ADD-R patients 20-25% have <u>Antisocial Personality
   Disorder</u> as well. Most of these individuals gave
   evidence of this behavior as children. Moreover, many
   ADDH patients go on to develop <u>alcoholism</u> and <u>substance
   abuse</u> problems as adults, although this is much more
   common in that subpopulation that has also developed a
   personality disorder.

2. The symptoms of the ADDH child most likely to last
   into adulthood include distractibility, restlessness,
   and emotional lability. Most also have a degree of
   low self-esteem.

3. In spite of continued symptoms, many ADD-R adults
   function satisfactorily in their jobs and interpersonal
   relationships.

4. A few ADD-R adults seem to respond well to antidepressants, although we do not yet know how to identify
   them ahead of time.

5. Many ADDH children have associated learning problems.
   Those problems generally persist into adulthood.

6. There is an increased incidence of ADDH, alcoholism,
   and antisocial and histrionic personality disorders in
   the biological parents of ADDH children.

PITFALLS:

1. It is easy to overlook this group of patients. Always
   consider ADD-R in the patient with a complex, varied,
   emotionally turbulent pattern of symptoms which have
   been present since childhood.

2. Do not conclude for emotional or political reasons (as some school systems have) that stimulants have no place in human pharmacotherapy.

REFERENCES

1. Amado H, Lustman PJ: Attention deficit disorders persisting in adulthood: A review. Comp Psychiatry 23:300-314, 1982.
2. Cantwell DP: Hyperactive children have grown up. Arch Gen Psychiatry 42:1026-1028, 1985.
3. Gittelman R, Mannuzza S, et al: Hyperactive boys almost grown up. Arch Gen Psychiatry 42:937-947, 1985.
4. Gomez RL, Janowsky D, et al: Adult psychiatric diagnosis and symptoms compatible with the hyperactive child syndrome: A retrospective study. J Clin Psychiatry 42:389-394, 1981.
5. Satterfield JH, Hoppe CM, Schell AM: A prospective study of delinquency in 110 adolescent boys with attention deficit disorder and 88 normal adolescent boys. Am J Psychiatry 139:795-798, 1982.
6. Tarter RE: Psychosocial history, minimal brain dysfunction and differential drinking patterns of male alcoholics. J Clin Psychology 38:867-873, 1982.
7. Weiss G, Hechtman L, et al: Psychiatric status of hyperactives as adults: A controlled prospective 15-year follow-up of 63 hyperactive children. J Amer Acad Child Psychiatry 24:211-220, 1985.
8. Wender PH, Reimherr FW, Wood D, Ward M: A controlled study of methylphenidate in treatment of attention deficit disorder, residual type, in adults. Amer J Psychiat 142:547-552, 1985.
9. Wood D, Wender PH, Reimherr FW: The prevalence of attention deficit disorder, residual type, or minimal brain dysfunction, in a population of male alcoholic patients. Am J Psychiatry 140:95-98, 1983.

CASE 43: Fred is a 20-year-old man living at home with his parents, much to their dismay. Although he has always been a loner, over the past four years he has become increasingly isolated and now seldom leaves his room.

The problem began in 10th grade with severe absenteeism: although he was a good student throughout junior high school, by his senior year he almost failed to be graduated because of missed days and failing grades. In the two years since finishing high school, he has resolutely resisted all inducements by his parents to either attend college or get a job: he has "retired" to his room.

He is brought today for a psychiatric interview by his mother since, according to her, he never would have come on his own. You attempt to obtain a history from him but each question is answered by his mother while Fred sits quietly and stares at the floor. His facial expression is "bland": he gives no visual signs of being depressed, excited, resentful, or agitated. Since he seems unwilling to talk and his mother is voluble, you decide to obtain additional history from her.

Fred had few friends as a child and virtually none as an adolescent. His peers throughout his school years teased him and considered him "weird," although his mother's best explanation was that he stood out by being too quiet. He has always been compliant around his parents, although over the last few years has become increasingly "stubborn" and testy when asked to become active outside the home. He has never used alcohol or drugs nor shown any obvious antisocial behavior.

Except for his shyness, his development has been normal. He has never been seen by a psychiatrist before although a high school counselor once suggested that he might need some "assertiveness training." His maternal grandmother died in the state mental hospital where she had spent many years due to her "hearing voices." His mother describes herself as having had several nervous breakdowns, although she has never been hospitalized. Fred's father had a long record of criminal offenses as a juvenile, two felony counts as an adult, but no emotional illness or substance abuse.

According to his mother, Fred is seldom anxious, is comfortable when meeting new people (in spite of his style during the interview) but does so only grudgingly, never complains of loneliness, and rarely becomes embarrassed or worried.

Upon his mother's insistence, Fred answers a few simple mental status questions which suggest that he is oriented, aware of the purpose of his visit, and reasonably intelligent. While continuing to "talk to the floor," he denies any problems and states that he wishes to leave. Although his speech is clear, his memory intact, and his performance on serial sevens and simple calculations flawless, he adds nothing to the interview spontaneously. He denies having hallucinations or delusions. Throughout the interview he is "distant" and never smiles.

You have concluded at this point that the patient probably suffers from a schizoid personality disorder and are about to bring the interview to a close but decide to make an attempt to talk to Fred without his mother present. When she has left the room, you tell him that he may go home if he answers just a few of your questions more fully.

CLINICAL CLUE:

Fred again denies hallucinations or delusions but when asked if he has ever had "mystical experiences," he replies that he ought to have since he is a wizard and a prophet. He then relates an elaborate delusional system in which he is the nerve center for the civilized world and can influence distant events by "pure thought." He notes that he hadn't mentioned this before because his mother considers these ideas silly and becomes upset when he talks about them.

QUESTIONS:

1. Why is the primary diagnosis <u>not</u> schizoid personality disorder?

2. Construct a differential diagnosis.

3. What is the correct diagnosis?

4. What was the patient's mother trying to hide by not telling the whole story?

5. What is the likelihood that Fred will improve significantly with antipsychotic medication?

ANSWERS:

1.   Although the patient has many of the characteristics
      of schizoid personality disorder such as indifference
      to praise or criticism, emotional aloofness, and a
      paucity of close friendships, he also has the positive
      symptom of bizarre ideas or delusions that immediately
      eliminates schizoid PD as the primary diagnosis.

2.   Young adults with borderline intellectual functioning
      occasionally will respond to a confusing and hostile
      world with withdrawal, however normal grades through
      junior high school argue against a low IQ in this case
      (although specific testing is desirable).
          A slow dementing process can produce altered
      behavior, isolation, and strange ideas. However, in a
      young person you would expect accompanying neurological
      symptoms. Moreover, a brief mental status examination
      in this patient found no evidence of dementia.   A
      careful physical and neurological examination is called
      for.
          Schizotypal personality disorder may present with
      withdrawal and peculiar thinking, however the odd
      ideas don't reach the level of delusions.
          Social phobia, separation anxiety disorder, and
      avoidant disorder of adolescence are all possibilities
      in an individual who is housebound and who avoids
      people and social contact. However, these conditions
      are characterized by anxiety and emotional distress
      when in certain situations such as when around others
      or when forced to leave the "safety" of home and
      family. Fred, on the other hand, preferred to remain
      at home but was comfortable in almost any situation.
          Patients with dysthymic disorder or major depres-
      sion may be quiet and withdrawn but, unlike Fred, they
      usually look depressed and will admit to feelings of
      sadness.

3.   Schizophrenia, Paranoid Type (DSM-III 295.3).   The
      deteriorating course, marked delusional ideas, and
      family history of a chronic psychotic illness all
      suggest that schizophrenia is the proper diagnosis.
      Although his delusional ideas were not overtly para-
      noid, systematized grandiose delusions result in the
      same diagnostic outcome by DSM-III standards.

4.   Initially it appeared that Fred's mother was defending
      against an awareness of the severity of her son's
      illness by failing to recognize that his strange ideas
      were more than "just foolishness." With time, however,
      it became clear that she had genuine difficulty appre-

ciating just how bizarre his ideas were: first degree relatives of patients with schizophrenia occasionally have altered perceptions and idiosyncratic thinking of their own without suffering overtly from schizophrenia.

5. Slim. Fred has most of the predictors of a poor outcome: a family history of schizophrenia, onset at an early age, no precipitating stress to his current episode, an absence of confusion or emotional features, prominent negative symptoms, and poor premorbid social functioning. His prognosis is poor and his course likely to be chronic.

PEARLS:

1. Do a careful mental status exam, even in "open and shut" cases.

2. The likelihood that Fred's only sister will develop schizophrenia sometime during her life is 10% (compared to approx. 1% in the general population).

3. Early evidence that a thinking disorder may be developing includes symptoms like difficulty keeping thoughts organized, wandering attention, rumination, preoccupations, inability to relax, difficulty planning ahead, and rambling and circumstantial speech.

PITFALLS:

1. Do not make the mistake of failing to interview a patient alone, when possible, no matter how clear and definite the information provided by a third party.

REFERENCES

1. Easson WM: The early manifestations of adolescent thought disorder. J Clin Psychiat 40:469-475, 1979.
2. Fish B: Neurobiological antecedents of schizophrenia in children. Arch Gen Psychiat 34:1297-1313, 1977.
3. Fowler RC, Tsuang MT, Cadoret RJ: Psychiatric illness in the offspring of schizophrenics. Comp Psychiat 18:127-134, 1977.
4. Grinker RR, Holzman PS: Schizophrenic pathology in young adults. Arch Gen Psychiat 28:168-175, 1973.
5. MacCrimmon DJ, Cleghorn JM, et al: Children at risk for schizophrenia. Arch Gen Psychiat 38:671-674, 1980.
6. Millon TM: Disorders of Personality. New York, John Wiley & Sons, 1981.
7. Rosenthal D, Kety SS: The Transmission of Schizophrenia. Oxford, Pergamon Press, 1968.

THE RESTLESS REALTOR

<u>CASE 44:</u> A psychiatric resident is called at midnight to see a patient who had been admitted to the neurology service for a seizure work-up. The neurology resident reports that the patient "seemed fine when we admitted him this afternoon. He didn't feel like eating dinner and seemed a little depressed, but in the last three hours he has become more and more anxious. We've talked to him and given him a sleeping pill (Halcion 0.25 mg), but nothing seems to calm him down."

A quick chart review reveals the patient to be a 52-year-old divorced realtor who had been discovered by a colleague three days ago in what appeared to be a grand mal seizure. Today he was admitted for a complete diagnostic work-up. There was no past or family history of seizures. He claimed to be in excellent health, although the coworker who accompanied him to the doctor's office at the time of the seizure had disclosed that he had called in sick "5 or 6 times" in the last month and that he had recently made two major errors that may result in dismissal from his job. Also, he had seemed more depressed and temperamental since his divorce two years ago.

The resident examines the patient and finds him crying, shaking, and repeatedly wailing "I'll never get to sleep. I can't take it anymore." He cannot say how he feels and has no idea what is wrong. On physical examination he is diaphoretic and hyperreflexic with a pulse of 130, blood pressure of 150/100, and temperature of 101.1°F. He has bruises on his head and right arm. The nurse who has been attending him comments that he looks like a patient she had last week with a "rapidly progressive infection." As the resident leaves the room, the nurse calls out, "He's having another seizure!"

LABORATORY CLUES:

Albumin 3.0 (nl = 3.8-5.0 gm%)
Direct bilirubin 0.6 (nl = 0.0-0.3 mg%)
Total bilirubin 3.0 (nl = 0.0-1.0 mg%)
SGOT 150 (nl = 1-51 IU/L)
LDH 400 (nl = 112-247 IU/L)
SGPT 100 (nl = 4-46 IU/L)

QUESTIONS:

1.   What is probably wrong with this patient?

2.   Name five medical complications associated with this disorder.

3.   What organic mental disorders are associated with this problem?

4.   Would the drug disulfiram be useful in the long-term management of this patient? By what biochemical mechanism does it work?

ANSWERS:

1. The most likely diagnosis is alcohol withdrawal in an alcohol-dependent person, though barbiturate/tranquilizer withdrawal would produce a similar picture. Hypoglycemia or diabetic ketoacidosis might also be considered, but the patient's age, social history, present illness, physical examination and laboratory data are most suggestive of alcohol dependence and withdrawal. It is likely that his recent work trouble and temperament changes relate to alcohol. His ex-wife was later contacted by phone. She confirmed his chronic heavy drinking and related that their divorce was largely based on his alcohol abuse.

    Ten percent of alcohol users experience significant alcohol-related problems and 20-50% of medical/surgical hospital admissions are in some way related to drinking. On admission, many deny or "forget to mention" their alcohol abuse and cases similar to this one, in which unexpected withdrawal begins after hospital admission, are commonplace. Whether recognized or not, alcoholic patients may be found in every medical practice.

    The DSM-III diagnosis of Alcohol Dependence requires pathological use or impaired social/occupational functioning secondary to alcohol, as well as tolerance and withdrawal. Pathological use may take many forms: daily need for alcohol in order to function adequately, inability to stop, binges, blackouts, drinking non-beverage alcohol, drinking more than a fifth a day, and repeated efforts to control alcohol use. Impaired social/occupational functioning may consist of physical violence while intoxicated, missing work, loss of job, arrests for intoxication, alcohol-related traffic accidents, or alcohol-related arguments and difficulties with family or friends. Tolerance consists of either the need for increased amounts of a substance to achieve the same effect or diminished effect with the same amount. Withdrawal symptoms, as in this patient, commonly come on 8-24 hours after the last drink. Early symptoms may consist of mild tremor, anorexia, insomnia, irritability, depression, anxiety, and weakness. Untreated, the symptom complex generally intensifies and progresses to coarse tremor, diaphoresis, hypertension, tachycardia, low-grade fever, disorientation and memory disturbance, with the possibility of progression to seizures, hallucinations, and delirium ("DTs").

2. Cirrhosis, neuropathy, seizures, gastritis, delirium tremens, Korsakoff's psychosis, myopathy, pancreatitis, and accidents.

3. Alcohol intoxication, alcohol idiosyncratic intoxication, alcohol withdrawal, alcohol withdrawal delirium (DTs), alcohol hallucinosis, alcohol amnestic disorder (Korsakoff's syndrome), and alcoholic dementia. Of these seven disorders, the first two do not imply either chronic or prolonged alcohol use. The remaining five, however, only occur after prolonged and excessive alcohol use.

4. The use of disulfiram (Antabuse) in the long-term management of alcoholism is a topic that after more than 30 years still is controversial. Most treatment programs do use disulfiram and cite a recent study showing twice as many abstinent patients in the disulfiram group, in addition to fewer work absences and more consistent treatment follow-up. Patient motivation and compliance are important factors in this treatment choice. Disulfiram alone (without additional therapies) is strongly discouraged.
    Disulfiram inactivates aldehyde dehydrogenase in the liver, blocking the regular route of alcohol metabolism and resulting in accumulation of acetaldehyde. Even small amounts of alcohol such as that absorbed through the skin from a cologne can cause acetaldehyde poisoning with symptoms of hypotension, nausea, malaise, dizziness, flushing, blurred vision, palpitations, or numbness. The most severe complication, hypotension, has resulted in death.

PEARLS:

1. Body temperatures over about $102^{\circ}F$ during withdrawal are generally secondary to a concomitant infection.

2. The most common symptoms associated with alcohol abuse/dependence are those of personal and family concern, while the most rare are job loss, DTs, and hospitalization.

3. A composite MMPI of a study group of alcoholics indicated personality characteristics centering around immaturity, dependency, resentment, excessive self-interest, and irresponsibility.

4. Anxiety, depression, dependency and sociopathy may be the result and not the cause of alcohol dependence.

5. Adoption studies have shown the risk of alcoholism to be elevated fourfold in the offspring of alcoholics adopted at birth and raised without contact with their biological parents. Environmental influences should

not be discounted, though genetics and biology undoubt-edly contribute to the development of alcoholism.

6. About 1/3 of men recovering from alcoholism find a new life partner - someone they have not injured in the past.

7. In males, secondary alcoholism is associated most frequently with antisocial personality disorder and in females with recurrent depression.

8. The majority of alcoholics suffer from some degree of cognitive dysfunction. Abstinence may ameliorate the impairment but complete recovery is rare.

9. Low serum magnesium levels have been associated with increased seizure risk during alcohol withdrawal. Many physicians administer magnesium sulfate routinely during the first few days of detoxification, though this practice is refuted by others.

PITFALLS:

1. The belief that alcoholism is simply a symptom of un-happy early life, family discord, and personality dis-order is incorrect.

2. The medical profession to often deals with the problem of alcoholism by denial (eg, ignoring even obvious signs of its presence in patients) and therapeutic nihilism (believing that it is basically untreatable).

3. Controlled social drinking does occur in a very few alcoholics but is not an appropriate treatment goal for most.

4. To date, no effective means have been developed to prevent alcoholism in groups at risk, however, it is predicted that future emphasis will increasingly center on prevention rather than tertiary treatment.

TRIVIA:

In the 1930's, electrical aversion (pairing painful electrical shocks with the sight, taste, and smell of alcoholic drinks) was used as a treatment for alcohol-ism by the Soviet physician, Kantorovich. He reported a 70% recovery rate, however, the technique has since been proven ineffective.

REFERENCES

1. American Psychiatric Association Task Force on Nomen-
    clature and Statistics: Diagnostic and Statistical
    Manual of Mental Disorders, 3rd ed. (DSM-III). Amer
    Psychiatric Association, Washington, DC, 1980.
2. Armor DJ, Polich JM, Stambul HB: Alcoholism and treat-
    ment. New York, John Wiley & Sons, 1978.
3. Grinspoon L: Psychiatry Update, Vol. III. Washington,
    DC, American Psychiatric Press, 1984.
4. Helzer JE, et al: The extent of long-term moderate
    drinking among alcoholics discharged from medical and
    psychiatric treatment facilities, NEJM 312:1678, 1985.
5. Schuckit MA: Alcoholism and genetics: Possible biolog-
    ical mediators. Biol Psychiat 15:437-447, 1980.
6. Vaillant GE: The Natural History of Alcoholism. Cam-
    bridge, MA, Harvard University Press, 1983.

CASE 45: Mrs. B, a 45-year-old legal secretary and mother of two, is brought to a psychiatrist's office by her concerned husband. He had called asking for an appointment and, when given a time 10 days in the future, remarked that he "didn't think she could wait that long." She was seen that afternoon on an emergency basis.

Mrs. B was dressed in wrinkled and slightly soiled clothing. Her hair was carelessly combed and there was a faint body odor about her. Her face was drawn and expressionless. She was helped by her husband into the office where she sat motionless, staring at the floor and occasionally sighing audibly. She said nothing unless asked a simple direct question. Even then her answers were delayed, spoken slowly, and of a droning, monotonous quality. A portion of the interview went as follows:

Dr. R:	What's the trouble that brings you in?
Mrs. B:	I don't care about anything.
Dr. R:	What do you mean?
Mrs. B:	(no response).
Dr. R:	You look sad.
Mrs. B:	Yes...not sad...just nothing.
Dr. R:	How long have you been like this?
Mrs. B:	About three weeks...getting worse.
Dr. R:	Has anything like this ever happened to you before?
Mrs. B:	No.
Dr. R:	How's your appetite?
Mrs. B:	No appetite.
Dr. R:	Have you lost weight these three weeks?
Mrs. B:	I don't know...maybe 10 or 12 lbs.
Dr. R:	How's your sleeping?
Mrs. B:	Bad. I wake up every morning about three and just lay there.
Dr. R:	Do you feel bad about anything?
Mrs. B:	Everything...I wish I were dead.

Mr. B is interviewed next. He relates that they have been married 26 years and she has never been like this before. The trouble seemed to begin about a month ago - she was too tired to go boating, "her favorite thing." "Gradually she has withdrawn. She doesn't want to see anybody, just wants to rest but I never see her sleeping. I force her to eat. I guess I panicked yesterday when she said she wanted to die."

As far as is known, she is in good medical health and uses neither alcohol, drugs, nor prescription medicines.

LABORATORY CLUE:

A dexamethasone suppression test (DST) was performed. One milligram of dexamethasone was administered at 11:00 PM. Blood cortisol determinations were made just prior to the dexamethasone dose and then the next day at 8 AM, 4 PM, and 10 PM. Results were as follows (in $\mu g\%$ of cortisol):

11 PM (pre-dexamethasone) —	17.5
8 AM —	6.8
4 PM —	12.5
10 PM —	14.8

(The test is abnormal if any of the post-dexamethasone cortisol determinations are greater than 4 $\mu g\%$.)

QUESTIONS:

1. What is the diagnosis?

2. Her speech and body movements are slowed. What term describes this symptom?

3. What is the biogenic amine hypothesis of affective disorders?

4. What was learned from the dexamethasone suppression test?

5. Name five medications which can cause serious depression as a side effect.

ANSWERS:

1. <u>Major Depression</u>, single episode, with melancholia
    (DSM-III, 296.23). Depressive disorder is the most
    common serious psychiatric disturbance. About 15% of
    the population will have at least one severe depression
    during their lifetime. Mrs. B's symptoms and presen-
    tation squarely meet the DSM-III criteria for major
    depression. However, some thought should be given to
    other possibilities such as depression secondary to
    drugs or medical illness. These seem unlikely but
    should always be considered. Dementias and schizo-
    phrenia can present with depressive symptomatology,
    but the premorbid history and rapid onset make these
    possibilities remote. Major depression is generally
    distinguished from dysthymic disorder by its distinct
    point of onset and clear demarcation between the
    depressed and premorbid behavior. The dysthymic dis-
    order, by contrast, has a vague and gradual onset, is
    less severe, and is more chronic (more than two years
    by DSM-III criteria).
        In DSM-III the term "melancholia" is used to
    refer to depressions characterized by symptoms such as
    early morning awakening, anorexia, weight loss, exces-
    sive guilt, marked psychomotor retardation or agita-
    tion, and/or a regular diurnal variation with symptoms
    worse in the morning. This condition has also been
    termed "endogenous depression."

2. "Psychomotor retardation" refers to the general slow-
    ing of mind and body which often accompanies severe
    depression. In the extreme, one can become totally
    mute and immobile. Less severe indications include
    slow speech, delayed speech (long pauses before answer-
    ing), no initiation of communication, monotonous tone,
    poverty of speech (markedly decreased quantity), and
    slowed laborious body movement. Also possible in
    severe depression is "psychomotor agitation." This is
    often manifested by nervous pacing, hand-wringing,
    restlessness, pressured speech, pulling at or rubbing
    clothes or other objects, and outbursts of shouting.
    "Retarded depression" and "agitated depression" are
    terms commonly used to refer to these conditions.

3. The biogenic amine hypothesis holds that some depres-
    sive disorders are secondary to an absolute or rela-
    tive deficiency of central nervous system neurotrans-
    mitters (particularly norepinephrine and serotonin),
    and that likewise manias may be associated with such
    neurotransmitter excesses. Even proponents of this

theory recognize it as an oversimplification of what is more likely an extremely complex biological system.

4. In the early 1980's it was discovered that about 70% of people with a major depression show an abnormal response to a dexamethasone challenge. The test has limited value in that there are often false negatives and many drugs and medical conditions interfere (such as carbamazepine, amphetamines, phenytoin, phenobarbital, meprobamate, alcohol withdrawal, pregnancy, Cushing's disease, hypopituitarism, Addison's disease, etc). In addition, non-suppression has been reported in other psychiatric disorders such as anorexia nervosa, bulimia, dementia, and obsessive-compulsive disorder. The test has been reported to be useful in differentiating schizophrenia from depression in difficult cases and in predicting response to antidepressant therapy. It has been reported that if a depressed patient has an abnormal DST that continues as abnormal during the antidepressant treatment, the patient will probably relapse if the treatment is discontinued.
    An abnormal DST was certainly not necessary to make the diagnosis in Mrs. B's case, however, it does help confirm this impression and underscores the seriousness of her condition.

5. Antihypertensives (reserpine, alpha-methyldopa, propranolol, guanethidine, hydralazine, clonidine)
    Corticosteroids (cortisone)
    Hormones (estrogen, progesterone)
    Antiparkinsonian agents (levodopa, amantadine)
    Chemotherapeutic agents (vincristine, vinblastine)

PEARLS:

1. Major depression can be superimposed on a chronic minor affective disorder such as dysthymic disorder. This state has been termed "double depression."

2. The incidence of depression is inversely related to social class.

3. Major depression is more common in women than men (about 2:1), whereas bipolar disorder is equally common.

4. Insomnia and anorexia are more common in major depression than hypersomnia and hyperphagia.

5. The prevalence of depression increases with age.

6.   Single and divorced persons are more likely to have depression than those who are married.

7.   Over 50% of patients who experience a single episode of major depression will eventually have another.

8.   Generally, people with recurrent major depressions return to their premorbid level of functioning between episodes. Some (20-30%) follow a chronic course showing increasing impairment between episodes.

PITFALLS:

1.   The widely held belief that the incidence of depression increases during the menopausal years is untrue.

2.   Stressful life events are neither a necessary nor sufficient cause for depression. Depressions of all types develop without life precipitants and conversely all life stresses are not followed by depression. However, marital, parental, and job stresses are most consistently linked to depression.

TRIVIA:

1.   The first system of psychiatric diagnosis was that formulated by Hippocrates in about 400 B.C. Two of his six diagnostic categories were mania and melancholia.

2.   An excellent novel dealing with the development and course of a major depression is The Bell Jar by Sylvia Plath.

REFERENCES

1.   American Psychiatric Association Task Force on Nomenclature and Statistics: Diagnostic and Statistical Manual of Mental Disorders, 3rd ed. (DSM-III). Amer Psychiatric Association, Washington, DC, 1980.
2.   Bowden CL: Current treatment of depression. Hosp & Com Psychiat 36:1192-1200, 1985.
3.   Costello CG: Social factors associated with depression: A retrospective community study. Psychol Med 12:329-339, 1982.
4.   Fava GA, et al: Treatment responses in 1^O and 2^O melancholia: A preliminary report. J Clin Psychiat 46:332-334, 1985.
5.   Garver DL, Davis JM: Biogenic amine hypothesis of affective disorders. Life Sci 24:383-394, 1979.

6. Hirschfeld RMA, Cross CK: Epidemiology of affective
    disorders: Psychosocial risk factors. Arch Gen Psychiat
    39:35-46, 1982.
7. Klerman GL: Overview of affective disorders. In Kaplan
    HJ, Freedman AM, Sadock BJ, Comprehensive Textbook of
    Psychiatry, 3rd Ed., Baltimore, Williams & Wilkins,
    1980.
8. Plath S: The Bell Jar. London, Faber and Faber, 1963.
9. Weissman MM, Merikangas KR, et al: Understanding the
    clinical heterogeneity of major depression using
    family data. Arch Gen Psychiat 43:430-434, 1986.

CASE 46:   The police bring a 32-year-old man to your office in shackles. They refuse your request to remove the hand- and legcuffs although they allow you to interview this individual in private.

He has been brought from the county jail where he is awaiting trial on charges of having molested a 7-year-old boy. Apparently his attorney is attempting to establish that a "serious mental illness" was responsible for his client's behavior. You have been retained as an "objective expert witness" by the county attorney's office which is prosecuting the case.

The defendant is pleasant, cooperative (he has been so instructed by his attorney), and willing to answer all your questions. A brief mental status examination is normal.

He had been arrested four weeks ago, after a child he had molested reported the incident to his parents. The defendant, who lived alone, had struck up friendships with several of the children who lived in his neighborhood. Moreover, he was well known to the parents in his apartment house as a "nice guy" who was always ready to help look after their children if they were detained at work or had to run to the store. He even had developed a romantic liaison with a divorced woman nearby, the mother of three young sons.

On the day of his arrest, he had invited a boy into his apartment by promising to show him his new video game. They played that game for a while, then shifted gradually to a variant of "you show me yours and I'll show you mine." The boy was given toys ("prizes") for taking off more clothes than the defendant, and then for "inspecting" him and allowing himself to be inspected once disrobed. The result was an episode of genital fondling during which the boy became acutely uncomfortable but was not harmed physi- cally. Sometime during the fondling, the defendant covert- ly masturbated. After that he brought the episode to a close and sent the boy home. The mother asked about the collection of new toys, heard the story, and called the police.

This episode is but one in a long series of molests by this man extending over the past 7 years. He has been sexually aroused by young boys since adolescence but has acted on those impulses only recently. He estimates that he has molested several dozen boys of ages 5 - 11 and has approached many more. He has no interest in girls, younger children, boys once they have developed secondary sexual characteristics, or adult women. (He was married briefly but supported that relationship sexually by fantasizing about young boys during intercourse.) He has never been (as far as we know) aggressive or violent with the children he has molested.

He describes having been interested in children and their welfare for as long as he can remember. He has been a boy scout leader and a member of Big Brothers. However, he frequently has used those associations to gain access to children. He has a college education and works as an accountant. He has not had close relationships outside of his family but generally has been well liked by those with whom he has worked.

SOCIOCULTURAL OBSERVATION:

> Upon returning him to the police at the conclusion of the interview, one of the officers comments: "I hope you aren't going to say anything good about this bastard."

QUESTIONS:

1.   What is the diagnosis?

2.   What causes this condition?

3.   Can this condition be treated successfully?

4.   What is the effect of a molest on a child?

5.   How do you explain the reaction of the police?

ANSWERS:

1.   <u>Pedophilia</u> (DSM-III, 302.20). These individuals become sexually aroused by immature children. Usually they lose interest once a child passes into adolescence (and thus they should be differentiated from those adults who become sexually involved with physically mature teenagers).

   Most pedophiles are interested exclusively in either males (<u>homosexual pedophilia</u>) or females (<u>heterosexual pedophilia</u>) but a few are aroused by both sexes. Most are males in their 20's or 30's but a few are older. Often they are fond of children, as well as being sexually attracted to them, and thus donate their time to child-oriented charity activities. (However, for some the only reason for such participation is to be exposed to children.)

   Few pedophiles are violent, being content with "seducing" the child with affection and gifts, followed by self-exposure and/or fondling. (However, this is not always the case. Shortly before this patient was seen, the same psychiatrist evaluated a 28-year-old homosexual pedophile for the court who, when he thought a boy's risk of reporting an incident of molest to his parents was too great, would kill the child. He was caught only after he had murdered several young boys.)

2.   We don't know. Many of these individuals were raised in turbulent homes, suggesting that abnormal childhood experiences and upbringing play a role. Others may have a "conditioned" eroticism based on early introduction to sexual activity with young playmates. Some pedophiles are uncomfortable around adults and only truly at ease when with children.

   Some recent studies suggest that there may be a biological component to pedophilia: one study showed that pedophiles had a marked elevation of luteinizing hormone (LH) in response to LHRH as compared to controls and patients with other types of sexual deviations.

3.   Yes, in some cases. Traditional treatments (most commonly 1-to-1 psychodynamic psychotherapy) have been notoriously unsuccessful. However, more effective treatment methods are now available that can change many pedophiles. Most noteworthy has been the application of several behavioral techniques that focus on at least four different areas simultaneously:
   A. Decreasing <u>deviant sexual arousal</u> (eg, arousal to small boys by some pedophiles) using aversive

conditioning (eg, shock)

B. Increasing <u>appropriate sexual arousal</u> (eg, arousal of males to adult females) by such techniques as coupling adult erotic material with masturbation.

C. Improving <u>heterosocial skills</u> (eg, the skills involved in getting along with adults of the opposite sex) through direct training.

D. Modifying <u>gender role identity</u> (ie, the sense the patient has of being "truly male").

Such a comprehensive behavioral approach (see Barlow, 1974) has proven effective with a number of different types of paraphilias, including pedophiles.

A few pedophiles are aggressive, driven, and "hypersexual." Treatment of these individuals with antiandrogenic medication which lowers the levels of plasma testosterone (eg, medroxyprogesterone acetate) often will halt their sexual behavior, although it typically leaves their sexual orientation unchanged (ie, they have the same impulses but they don't act on them).

4. It varies. While most children are distressed, made anxious, experience school difficulties, or suffer from depression acutely following a single episode of molest, the majority show little effect long-term. On the other hand, long lasting problems frequently follow molestations which are either particularly violent or are repeated many times (often over months or years) before ceasing.

    In addition, the response to the molestation by important adults (parents, police) influences the outcome. The more "terrible" it is made to seem to the child (eg, lengthy interviews by the police, vocal soul-searching by the parents), the more likely there is to be an unfavorable outcome.

5. Not only did these police officers (as do most adults) feel that sexual abuse of children is the most heinous of crimes, but they had also been involved over many months in the search for a "child killer" in the same town and thus allowed their strong feelings about him to generalize to all pedophiles.

PEARLS:

1. Pedophilia seems to run in families. Whether this reflects "nature" or "nurture" is as yet unknown.

2. Because of the social prohibition against the sexual approach of children, some "pedophiles" never act on their impulses but, rather, live their sexual life in fantasy only.

3. Although the statistics are unreliable, best estimates are that 15-30% of children have some sort of sexual experience with an adult at some time.

4. Emotionally insecure or love-deprived children are at increased risk of molestation since they are often receptive to adults offering affection.

PITFALLS:

1. Most studies of pedophilia have been done with people who have been arrested. Since some experts estimate that less that 5% of pedophiliacs ever come to the attention of the law, the data about pedophilia probably is inaccurate and reflects the more disturbed and extreme end of the spectrum.

2. Do not mistake as pedophiles those adults who molest children, not because of deviant sexual arousal, but because of certain conditions which alter impulse control: eg, psychosis, intoxication, retardation, dementia. The treatment is quite different.

TRIVIA:

Several British pedophiliacs have formed an organization known as Paedophilia Information Exchange (PIA) which attempts to present pedophilia in a positive light as a legitimate sexual preference.

REFERENCES

1. Abel GG, Blanchard EB: The role of fantasy in the treatment of sexual deviation. Arch Gen Psychiat 30:467-475, 1974.
2. Bancroft J: Human Sexuality and Its Problems. London, Churchill Livingstone, 1983.
3. Barlow DH: The treatment of sexual deviation: Toward a comprehensive behavioral approach. In Calhoun K, Adams H, Mitchell K, eds., Innovative Treatment Methods in Psychopathology. New York, John Wiley & Son, 1974.
4. Berlin FS, Meinecke CF: Treatment of sex offenders with antiandrogenic medication: Conceptualization, review of treatment modalities, and preliminary findings. Am J Psychiat 138:601-607, 1981.
5. Cordoba OA, Chapel JL: Medroxyprogesterone acetate antiandrogen treatment of hypersexuality in a pedophiliac sex offender. Am J Psychiat 140:1036-1039, 1983.

6. Gaffney GR, Berlin FS: Is there hypothalamic-pituitary-gonadal dysfunction in paedophilia?. Brit J Psychiat 145:657-660, 1984.

7. Gaffney GR, Lurie SF, Berlin FS: Is there familial transmission of pedophilia? J Nerv Ment Dis 172:546-548, 1984.

8. Hayes SC, Brownell KD, Barlow DH: Heterosocial-skills training and covert sensitization: Effects on social skills and sexual arousal in sexual deviants. Behav Res Ther 21:383-392, 1983.

9. Money J: Paraphilias: Phenomenology and classification, Amer J Psychotherapy 38:164-179, 1984.

THE ORGAN RECITAL

<u>CASE 47</u>:   You are asked to provide a psychiatric consulta-
tion on Mrs. W, a 34-year-old, white, thrice-married,
mother of two, who has been admitted to the medical service
with a chief complaint of "headaches and vomiting."   This
is her sixth hospitalization in 8 years for diagnostic
studies.   Three other hospital stays during this time had
been for a cholecystectomy, hysterectomy, and exploratory
laparotomy.   Past diagnoses recorded in the chart were
"adhesions," migraine headaches, "colitis," hypoglycemia,
and gastroenteritis.
     You enter her room and find her having a lively visit
with a younger sister.   They are reviewing the latest issue
of a fashion magazine.   She is dressed in a frilly purple
nightgown with gold trim, has long lavender fingernails,
and copious eye makeup.   Her gestures and facial expressions are engaging (if not exaggerated) and she immediately
impresses you as outgoing and pleasant.   In fact, she is
rather attractive and fun to talk with.   When you introduce
yourself as a psychiatrist she excuses her sister and asks
if you would like to see the fashions that she has selected
from the magazine, "Maybe that will help you get to know
me."
     Ninety minutes later you have obtained a vague and
complex medical history which appears to begin in her young
teen years with stomachaches.   Menstrual complaints, including extreme pain and incapacitation, dominated her
adolescence and eventually led to the hysterectomy at age
29.   She characterizes her headaches as "always there.
They never go away or let up.   It's like a hot poker is
stuck through my forehead."   With regard to the vomiting
she complains, "I wretch until blood comes up.   It started
with my last pregnancy (8 years ago).   I vomited the whole
nine months and it just keeps getting worse."   Other
complaints include dizziness, weakness, abdominal pain,
diarrhea, dysparunia, shortness of breath, genital burning
pain, racing heart, painful urination, fainting spells, and
blurred vision.   Near the end of the interview she remarks,
"Would you like to do a physical?   I'm developing a cough."

OBSERVATIONAL CLUE:

          As you are about to leave the room her current
     husband arrives for a visit.   You observe an immediate
     change in her demeanor - she becomes sullen and pouty
     and asks for "a shot of something strong to take away
     the headache."   Minutes later from the nurses' station
     you hear her in a

rage shouting, "Why can't your mother stay another week. I'm certainly in no condition to care for the kids, the house, the neighbors, and you, and everything else!"

QUESTIONS:

1. What three terms could be used to diagnose this problem?

2. What does the term "secondary gain" refer to? Are there any indications of secondary gain in this case?

3. What clues do you have as to this person's personality?

4. What advice or treatment suggestions do you have for the internist who requested your opinion?

5. What is the prognosis?

ANSWERS:

1.   The terms "hysteria" and "Briquet's syndrome" (often
      used interchangeably) have been largely replaced by
      the DSM-III diagnosis of <u>somatization disorder</u>. This
      is one of the <u>somatoform disorders</u>: conditions in which
      physical symptoms mimicking medical illness have no
      apparent organic etiology but rather are based on
      psychological factors. (The term "somatization" refers
      to the use of the body (soma) for psychological pur-
      poses or personal gain.) The underlying emotional
      issues commonly involve relationships, psychological
      conflicts, and social or environmental problems. So-
      matization disorder is common, of early onset (before
      age 30), and chronic. The course is typically fluc-
      tuating, with spontaneous remissions and relapses - a
      year without medical attention is rare. Complaints
      invariably involve numerous organ systems and are pre-
      sented in a dramatic or vague style - usually as a
      part of a long and complex medical history.
          Such patients often come from troubled homes with
      alcoholic or sociopathic parents, show poor school and
      social adjustments, adolescent delinquency, unstable
      marriages, and multiple husbands who are themselves
      frequently alcoholic and/or sociopathic.

2.   "Secondary gain" refers to the "benefits" that come to
      an individual as a result of the illness. These
      commonly involve avoidance of undesirable responsibi-
      lities, gaining support, sympathy or attention, or
      obtaining disability payments. Mrs. W's behavior when
      her husband entered the room seemed to engender
      sympathy and may win her support and attention from
      him. Her rage about his mother not staying is cause
      to suspect secondary gain which relieves her of house-
      hold and child care responsibilities.
          The term "secondary loss" has been applied to the
      detriments that usually accompany secondary gains -
      such as loss of approval, loss of respect, and the
      social stigma attached to one with chronic complaints.

3.   Her presentation is:
      <u>Dramatic and emotional</u>: Note her description of various
          symptoms ("like a hot poker sticking through my
          forehead"), her exaggerated gestures and facial
          expressions, and her obvious overstatement and
          exaggeration of fact (the headaches are "always
          there. They never go away or let up." "I vomited
          the whole nine months.")
      <u>Narcissistic, seductive and exhibitionistic</u>: She is
          overdressed and overly made-up for the occasion

(a hospital inpatient). Her invitation to show you the fashions she has chosen for herself is egocentric and suggests preoccupying self-interest and desire for your admiration and praise. Her direct invitation for a physical exam is inappropriate and openly seductive.

Manipulative: She appears skilled in getting what she wants from people. In this short exam we have seen rage, moody/pouty temperament, engaging warmth, sympathy engendering, dramatic exaggeration, and seductiveness.

It is highly likely that her personality is histrionic - a condition often but not invariably associated with somatization disorder.

4.   Once the diagnosis has been established, a major consideration becomes protecting the patient from herself. The financial cost, morbidity and even mortality from invasive diagnostic procedures, unnecessary surgery, and inappropriate medication are significant issues which are usually best managed by a primary care physician. Psychiatric referral is usually derogated by the patient and the more physicians involved in ongoing care the greater the likelihood of manipulation and poor management. It is difficult at times to sort out what new symptoms and complaints warrant work-up and treatment. These patients are still subject to true physical disease and should not be denied appropriate care on the basis of the hysteria.

The use of medication is a particular problem. Huge supplies of various medications prescribed for doubtful indications is the rule. Drug dependence (especially to tranquilizers, narcotic analgesics, and hypnotics) is common in this group, as are impulsive overdoses and adverse drug-drug interactions. Medication should be used with caution and prescribed in small quantities. A good general rule is that objective findings rather than subjective complaints should determine the use of diagnostic procedures and medical/surgical treatments.

Communication with the family is helpful in obtaining an accurate history, minimizing manipulation, coordinating the management approach, and providing care for what is usually a troubled family. Psychotherapies based on abreaction or expression of "locked up" emotion are contraindicated. These patients are too extreme in this direction to begin with.

5.   A "cure" is unlikely. The disorder is refractory to change - patients usually follow a chronic fluctuating course and are never entirely free of symptoms. Concentrate on long-term management instead.

PEARLS:

1.   Somatization disorder is estimated to occur in 1-2% of the female population. It is rare in males.

2.   Family studies show an increased prevalence of alcoholism and hysteria in female relatives of hysterics and alcoholism and sociopathy in the male relatives and husbands. Some speculate that hysteria in women and sociopathy in men may be different expressions of the same underlying pathology.

3.   A major complication of somatization disorder is excessive and unnecessary surgery. One study found hysterics twice as likely to have had major surgery, 6 times as likely to have had minor surgery, and 7 times as likely to have had GYN surgery.

4.   The symptoms of somatoform disorders are not under voluntary control, as they are in factitious disorders or malingering.

PITFALLS:

1.   Do not confine your image of the somatization disorder patient to one who is young and seductive. Such patients grow old and follow-up studies have demonstrated that the symptom pattern remains stable.

2.   Do not look too harshly on those whose illness is "somatoform" (Judge not that ye be not judged). Of medical students, 70-80% become wrongly fearful or convinced that they have a disease at sometime during their medical education. This phenomenon - "medical student disease" - occurs with equal frequency during the four years of medical school and the illness "chosen" is generally one of a current patient or an illness currently being studied.

3.   The "somatoform" group of disorders does not include the "psychosomatic" diseases such as asthma, peptic ulcer disease, or ulcerative colitis. These disorders are likely multi-determined and involve genetic, environmental, and psychological factors.

TRIVIA:

      The direct cost of medical care for the somatoform disorders is estimated to be about $20,000,000,000 annually (U.S., 1980). This figure does not include disability payments or the value of work time lost, and seems especially wasteful when one realizes that most medical treatment directed toward psychological problems is ineffective.

REFERENCES

1. American Psychiatric Association Task Force on Nomenclature and Statistics: Diagnostic and Statistical Manual of Mental Disorders, 3rd ed. (DSM-III). Amer Psychiatric Association, Washington, DC, 1980.
2. Chodoff P: Hysteria in women. Am J Psychiat 139:545-551, 1982.
3. DeVaul RA, Faillace LA: Surgery-proneness: A review and clinical assessment. Psychosomat 21:295-299, 1980.
4. Ford CV: The Somatizing Disorders: Illness as a way of Life. New York: Elsevier Biomedical, 1983.
5. Morrison JR: Management of Briquets syndrome (hysteria). West J Med 128:482-487, 1978.
6. Murphy GE: Clinical management of hysteria. JAMA 247:2559-2564, 1982.
7. Torgersen S: Genetics of somatoform disorders. Arch Gen Psychiat 43:502-505, 1986.
8. Woods SM, Natterson J, Silverman J: Medical student's disease: Hypochondriasis in medical education. J Med Education 41:785-790, 1966.

CASE 48: A 32-year-old, unmarried woman was referred to the sleep clinic by her psychiatrist with the complaint of chronic insomnia. Her difficulty falling asleep at night has persisted over the past two years in spite of seemingly endless trials of benzodiazepines and thoroughgoing psychotherapy.

Recently, however, things have changed. Not only does it take her an hour or more to fall asleep but now she is waking up frequently throughout the night and seldom sleeps past 5:00 AM. Both she and her psychiatrist are frustrated.

She presents as a pleasant, polite, but very high-strung woman who is at her wits' end over her sleeping problem. "I've tried everything. So has Dr. Strong. This is the curse of my life. I haven't slept well for as long as I can remember but this past month has been unbelievable. I'm tired all the time. I can't get to sleep. I can't stay asleep. Nothing is working out for me." She then breaks into tears.

After she has composed herself, you inquire into her sleeping habits. She usually gets to bed by 10:00 PM, but work as a private duty nurse occasionally prevents that. For many years she would toss and turn for "hours" before falling asleep but then usually would wake rested. Over the past 3 months, however, she has been waking at night, has required minutes to an hour or more to fall back to sleep, and has felt "drugged" all day. She has had trials of Dalmane, Restoril, Halcion, Nembutal, and Seconal but none were effective for more than a week or two. She has tried biofeedback, meditation, and relaxation techniques but she "never caught on" to them. It's become such a problem that she has noticed herself in the middle of the day worrying about how she will get to sleep that night.

During the interview she shows herself to be tense, anxious, and concerned that her sleep problems will never be resolved. She feels that this is her personal "weak link" and is convinced that it has prevented her from accomplishing anything worthwhile, either professionally or socially. A formal mental status exam is unremarkable.

OBSERVATIONAL CLUE:

When asked what single thing most helps her fall asleep, she replied: "A stiff drink."

QUESTIONS:

1.   What does DIMS stand for?

2.   What is the cause of her insomnia?

3.   What do you make of her changing sleep pattern?

4.   Should she have a polysomnography exam?

5.   What treatment would you recommend?

ANSWERS:

1.   Disorders of Initiating and Maintaining Sleep. This
      is the new term for insomnia. Thus, insomnia is not
      just an inability to fall asleep but also a mixture of
      problems maintaining sleep.

2.   There is no single cause. As so often happens with
      chronic insomnia, the etiology becomes mixed and con-
      fused over time. The Association of Sleep Disorders
      Centers (ASDC) classification recognizes a number of
      different types of insomnia, including:
      Transient, situational insomnia - caused by intraper-
            sonal, interpersonal, or environmental stress and
            lasting until the stress improves (or no more
            than 3 weeks).
      Psychophysiological insomnia -- patients become "condi-
            tioned" to the expectation that they won't be
            able to sleep, dwell on it, and such excessive
            concern thus becomes a self-fulfilling prophecy.
      Insomnia of psychiatric disorders - psychiatric condi-
            tions frequently associated with poor sleep
            include depression, anxiety disorder and panic,
            obsessive-compulsive disorder, psychosis, and
            hypochondriasis.
      Alcohol and drug related insomnia - chronic use of
            alcohol and hypnotic/sedatives produces fractured
            sleep as does use of stimulants, hallucinogens,
            opiates, thyroid, and some chemotherapeutic drugs.
      Respiratory impairment insomnia - conditions of sleep
            apnea and pulmonary hypoventilation can produce
            chronic insomnia.
      Nocturnal myoclonus and "restless legs" syndrome -
            both of these distinct but poorly understood
            conditions can impair sleep, even though the
            patient may not be aware of their presence.

      This patient had at least four factors contributing to
      her insomnia: (1) she was an anxious, driven person
      with a low tolerance for frustration; (2) she presum-
      ably had been "medicating" herself with alcohol (in
      fact, she had been drinking heavily over the preceding
      several months); (3) she had become clinically de-
      pressed; and (4) she had developed a conditioned
      negative expectation about her ability to fall asleep.
      Which of these factors, if any, started the ball
      rolling could no longer be determined, yet they were
      all playing a role in keeping it in motion.

3.   Anxiety, stress, and conditioning generally produce an
      insomnia characterized by difficulty falling asleep

(this patient's "lifelong" pattern), whereas depression and substance abuse tend to produce broken
sleep with frequent awakenings and early morning
arousal (the pattern she displayed with her worsening
insomnia over the several months prior to referral).
Thus, she probably became depressed, tried to treat
her depression and insomnia with alcohol, and ended up
with an altered and worsened sleeping problem.

4. Yes. Although sleep lab exams are not for everyone,
her picture was complicated enough and chronic enough
to warrant such a study. You would be looking for the
decreased REM latency and limited stage 3 and 4 sleep
found with depression as well as the frequent awakenings, decreased stage 3 and 4 and REM sleep, and increased beta sleep found in alcohol abuse.
Other conditions which may be unsuspected by the
patient but which are often clearly displayed by a
polysomnography study include sleep apnea, nocturnal
myoclonus, restless legs syndrome, and normal sleep.
In general, if insomnia has been present for months or
years and has been unresponsive to a variety of
sensibly chosen treatments, a lab study is indicated.

5. Treatment is twofold: psychological and pharmacological.

Psychological methods include psychotherapy for the
depression, addressing the alcohol abuse, searching
for any specific neurotic conflicts, investigating her
interpersonal style, etc. You should teach her
proper sleep hygiene: exercise regularly, wake at a
regular time each morning, keep busy during the day,
avoid heavy bedtime snacks, go to bed only when sleepy
generally avoid daytime naps, make the bedroom dark
and quiet, develop a "sleeping ritual" of several
things to do routinely before going to bed. Apply one
or more specific behavioral techniques: progressive
relaxation (when in bed, concentrate on relaxing one
muscle, then another, then back to the first, and so
on), meditation, biofeedback, paradoxical intention
(eg, tell her to go to bed and try not to sleep),
hypnosis, sleep restriction (restrict sleep to only a
few hours each night and then increase the time allowed
for sleep gradually).

For this patient, two types of medication may be
useful. If her depression appears clinically significant, a sedative antidepressant such as amitriptyline
may be used both for its antidepressant effect as well
as its short-term sedative effect. The use of a
hypnotic is more problematical. Short-acting (temaze-

pam, lorazepam, triazolam) and longer-acting (flurazepam) benzodiazepines are useful for treating brief insomnia but may not increase sleeping time in chronic forms. Even with transient insomnia, although hypnotics clearly lengthen sleep, there is question as to whether they improve functioning on the next day. At most, the use of hypnotics in chronic insomnia should be brief (one or two weeks), intermittent, and coordinated with psychotherapeutic efforts (eg, to help develop confidence that a new behavioral technique can be effective.

PEARLS:

1. Insomnia is the most common sleep complaint. Each year 35% of the population experiences a serious bout of it and 5% of the population takes sleeping pills for it.

2. The frequency of insomnia increases with age.

3. Almost 20% of the people who complain of chronic insomnia have normal sleep.

4. Some people are actually afraid to go to sleep at night (and with some reason) - more people die from natural causes at night than during the day.

5. Depression is the most common cause of serious, chronic insomnia.

6. In sleep laboratory populations (but not in the general clinic) hypersomnia is more common than insomnia.

7. Insomnia can come to dominate a person's life.

PITFALLS:

1. Don't assume that just because a person says she has insomnia that it is so.

2. Don't send every insomniac to the sleep lab. A good sleep and psychiatric history will provide clues to most important conditions.

REFERENCES

1. Coleman RM, Roffwarg HP, et al: Sleep-wake disorders based on a polysomnographic diagnosis. JAMA 247:997-1003, 1982.

2. Greenblatt DJ, Shader RI, Abernethy DR: Current status of benzodiazepines. NEJM 309:354-358, 1983.
3. Hauri PJ, Hayes B, et al: Effectiveness of a sleep disorders center: A 9-month follow-up. Am J Psychiat 139:663-666, 1982.
4. Kales A, Kales JD: <u>Evaluation and Treatment of Insomnia.</u> Oxford, Oxford Univ Pr, 1984.
5. Kales JD, Kales A, et al: Biopsychobehavioral correlates of insomnia. V. Clinical characteristics and behavioral correlates. Am J Psychiat 141:1371-6, 1984.
6. Mellinger GD, Balter MB, Uhlenhuth EH: Insomnia and its treatment. Arch Gen Psychiat 42:225-232, 1985.
7. Piccione P, Tallarigo R, et al: Personality differences between insomniac and non-insomniac psychiatry outpatients. J Clin Psychiat 42:261-263, 1981.

CASE 49: A friend from medical school is just beginning
his family practice in the city in which you have been
practicing for the past year. He calls to ask about
getting together for lunch. When you suggest a time two
weeks off, the tone of his voice drops, "I'd hoped to find
a time a little sooner." It appears that he is concerned
about something more than reminiscing over old times.

You meet at the restaurant a few days later, having
not seen each other for six years. After a few pleasant
moments remembering "the good old days," he takes on a more
serious tone. "When I set up my practice here, the first
thing I did was meet with several of the older established
doctors. I asked them for a few referrals to help get me
started and so far I've seen about 15 patients. Several
are really complicated. I actually think they referred me
their "crocks." There is a Mr. Samuels, 43 years old, who
has called me every day since I first saw him. He 'knows'
he has stomach ulcers, but nobody can find them. He's had
a dozen work-ups, takes about seven different medications,
complains all the time of pain, and thinks he's going to
get cancer. A Miss Thomas is only 27 and thinks she has
heart disease. She's always taking her pulse and wondering
if her heartbeat is 'regular enough.' She keeps noticing
'missed beats' and said to me absolutely seriously, 'If
it's heart disease, just tell me. I could live with that
easier than this game of nobody willing to admit it.' Her
mother gave her a blood pressure cuff for Christmas and she
carries it in her purse. I spent almost two hours last
week with a Mr. Jacobs. He told me every complaint he'd
ever had for the last 30 years. I thought we got along
fine. I even told him I didn't think anything was
seriously wrong and had some ideas that I thought could
help him get better. He called the next day so angry and
mean I didn't even know it was the same person at first.
He said he's going back to his old doctor.

"I'm in a real spot. I've seen these types before but
I could always get rid of them or put up with them for a
few months until I rotated to a new service. Now I'm
stuck. I can't send them back or accuse these doctors of
dumping on me. If I'm going to survive in this city, I've
got to work this out."

QUESTIONS:

1. What is most likely the problem with these three patients?

2. What factors appear to predispose one to develop "illness behavior?"

3. Should you offer to see these patients in consultation and possibly take over their treatment?

4. What was wrong with the way he handled Mr. Jacobs?

5. If you offer your friend some helpful suggestions, maybe he'll pay for lunch. What can you tell him?

ANSWERS:

1. Hypochondriasis. "The essential feature is a clinical picture in which the predominant disturbance is an unrealistic interpretation of physical signs or sensations as abnormal, leading to preoccupation with the fear or belief of having a serious disease. A thorough physical evaluation does not support the diagnosis of any physical disorder that can account for the physical signs or sensations or for the individual's unrealistic interpretation of them, although a coexisting physical disorder may be present. The unrealistic fear or belief of having a disease persists despite medical reassurance and causes impairment in social or occupational functioning" (DSM-III, p. 249).

2. Culture. Certain cultures appear to be more accepting of illness than others. For instance, college-age American Jews are more likely to see physicians, take medication, and be absent from life responsibilities when ill than white Protestants. A society that accepts physical illness but not emotional disorders favors somatic symptoms. Emotional symptoms are sometimes interpreted as showing weakness and inadequacy and to be "one's own fault." An overburdened housewife may win more sympathy and understanding by stomach pains, nausea, and weakness, than by anxiety, crying, irritability, and withdrawal.
    Inadequate social support system. A low level of social support (eg, living alone with no available family) correlates with increased use of medical services and has been shown to be a more potent variable than one's actual state of health.
    Life stress.
    Psychological resolution. Illness behavior is more likely when it can resolve personal or social problems. One might avoid unpleasant duties, personal responsibilities, blame for failure, sex, etc by being sick.
    Low self-reliance.

3. No. At least not at this point. Hypochondriacal patients generally refuse mental health referral and are not commonly seen by mental health professionals. They are usually offended by any suggestion that their fears or symptoms are unwarranted and interpret psychiatric referral as an opinion that the problems are "all in their head." If such a referral at this early stage does not drive the patient off, it would tend to establish an adversarial position and hamper the development of a therapeutic relationship.

4. It's hard to say with absolute certainty, but some
    things are suggested by the account presented. It was
    probably a mistake to minimize his complaints with the
    opinion that there was nothing "seriously wrong."
    Such patients often unconsciously tie much of their
    life's meaning, purpose, and importance to their ill-
    ness and suffering. The idea that their complaints
    are not substantial may be received as belittling and
    insulting. Also, the well-meaning optimism that he
    could help the patient get better may have been coun-
    terproductive. Such patients interface with the world
    largely through their physical complaints and worries.
    Their relationships often center around their symptoms.
    "Getting better" is commonly tied to being rejected
    and having no basis for interaction, friendship, and
    acceptance.

5. Hypochondriacal patients, as a rule, are best managed
    by primary care physicians. Their care should be
    viewed in terms of long-term management as opposed to
    cure. Most are not looking for cure and may even be
    threatened by the prospect.
        Establish a trusting relationship. Complete a
    thorough medical and personal history - even if it
    takes several visits. Time spent in this early phase
    will be well worth the effort in the long run. A
    physical exam and laboratory work-up should carefully
    exclude underlying disease but not be so extensive or
    esoteric as to reinforce the hypochondriacal complaints.
    Do not offer the patient new and undiscovered reasons
    for worry, mistrust, and doubt.
        Schedule regular appointments: an office visit
    should not end without the patient having another
    appointment. The request to "call for an appointment
    if the problem gets worse" or "drop back if you're not
    feeling better in a while" is essentially an invita-
    tion to develop new symptoms or "get worse" in order
    to return. Early on, visits may need to be frequent
    (eg, weekly) with the interval lengthening commensurate
    with the patient's level of trust. Respond to in-
    creasing complaints or more frequent phone calls by
    scheduling more frequent appointments.
        Expectations of cure expressed to the patient or
    assurances that the symptoms will be removed are
    contraindicated. A more neutral position is best -
    neither too optimistic nor pessimistic. One way to
    state this would be, "These are very complex symptoms
    and it may be that you will never be entirely free of
    them. But I'd like to help in the ways that I can.
    We'll hope to learn more about the problems as time
    goes on and find ways to minimize your suffering."

Any challenge of the symptoms or implication that "it's all in your head" would be counterproductive. In addition, the temptation to account for the patient's multiple symptoms by some minor physical or laboratory finding or to prescribe some innocuous medication "just to satisfy them" should be avoided. Such tactics only tend to reinforce and justify somatic preoccupation. (Patients with hypochondriasis that is secondary to depression may benefit from antidepressants.) Annoyance and irritation at the patient's ongoing symptoms will generally only kindle his anger and lead to even more intense symptoms or more difficult management problems.

A warm interest and positive regard should begin to communicate an acceptance of the patient that is not dependent on his having symptoms and complaints. Ideally, as the patient feels trust and acceptance, he will talk increasingly about personal and life issues, discover that his relationship with you is not dependent on his having physical complaints, and allow him to explore the emotions, stresses, relationships and other issues that underly the symptoms.

Group treatment (best referred to as a "Coping with Illness" group and held in the medical area of the clinic) has been shown to be cost effective, to increase psychological adjustment, decrease physical complaints, and decrease clinic visits.

PEARLS:

1. It has been estimated that 3-10% of physician visits are for hypochondriacal complaints.

2. Hypochondriasis commonly begins in adolescence but can occur at any subsequent age.

3. Hypochondriacal complaints are most frequently referable to the musculoskeletal, gastrointestinal, and central nervous systems.

4. Depression presenting with physical complaints rather than mood complaints has been termed "masked depression."

5. A study of consecutive patients reporting to a medical clinic determined that 43% had organic pathology, 13% had organic pathology plus significant psychological overlay, and 38% had no organic disease and only psychological problems (6% had no diagnosis).

6. Illness does not occur in a random pattern. One study found that about 50% of all illness occurs in only 25% of the population. Some experts postulate that those with a high frequency of illness have an impaired ability to adapt to life stresses and changing environments or circumstances.

PITFALLS:

1. Patients with somatoform disorders occupy a significant proportion of any physician's time, yet little attention is devoted to their diagnosis and treatment in most medical schools.

2. Patients whose illnesses do not conform to the usual medical diagnostic and treatment principles are often resented by their physicians.

3. Some hypochondriacal patients develop genuine organic disease as a side effect or complication of unjustified diagnostic and treatment interventions.

TRIVIA:

1. The term hypochondria (literally "beneath the cartilage") refers to that area of the upper abdomen just beneath the xiphoid process. This is the anatomic area which was believed to be the source of disease-causing humors.

2. In 18th Century England hypochondriasis (known as the "English Malady") was treated with spa vapors and regarded with pride as a condition of the civilized.

REFERENCES

1. Adler G: The physician and the hypochondriacal patient. NEJM 304:1394-1396, 1981.
2. American Psychiatric Association Task Force on Nomenclature and Statistics: Diagnostic and Statistical Manual of Mental Disorders, 3rd ed. (DSM-III). Amer Psychiatric Association, Washington, DC, 1980.
3. Barsky AJ, Wyshak G, Klerman GL: Hypochondriasis. Arch Gen Psychiat 43:493-500, 1986.
4. Brown HN, Valliant GE: Hypochondriasis. Arch Int Med 141:723-726, 1981.
5. Ford CV: The Somatizing Disorders: Illness as a Way of Life. New York, Elsevier Biomedical, 1983.
6. Kaplan HI, Sadock BJ: Comprehensive Textbook of Psychiatry, 4th ed. Baltimore, Williams & Wilkins, 1985.
7. McCranie EJ: Hypochondriacal neurosis. Psychsomat 20:11-15, 1979.

CASE 50: Mrs. G, 53 years old, presents for an appointment she made to discuss her son, Edward, a journeyman carpenter who at age 32 is still living at home and working only sporadically. He had been sickly as a child and "was babied": received constant attention, "got his own way," and commonly missed school for insignificant reasons. She confessed that, "Looking back we can see that we should have been more firm. But we were young, we didn't know any better, and we loved him so much. He finally finished high school, but didn't get a job until he was 20. He'd always say he wasn't ready yet. We wanted him to get out on his own, but we just couldn't kick him out. He's so polite and nice, we can't do anything to hurt him. It's starting to bother me, though. I fix all his meals and if he ever does get a job it's because I've found it and talked to the foreman. Once I even drove him to the job site and back every day for a month. My husband and I haven't been away alone together for over 20 years. We started talking about it at dinner last week. When we mentioned that we wanted to go alone, Edward couldn't eat anymore and went to his room. I feel so bad about hurting him, but we've just got to get away."

You ask to meet Edward and arrange an appointment for the next week. The following day you receive another phone call from Mrs. G. "Edward is in the hospital. My husband got mad at him last night for the first time and told him we were going on the trip whether he liked it or not. This morning we found him on the floor. He can't walk. The ambulance driver thought it was a stroke." You call a neurologist colleague who admitted Edward to the hospital. He reports, "Everything is normal - routine lab, thyroid, CPK, neurological exam, and EMG. We got him up to try to walk. He'd lurch and zigzag, then fall to someone who could catch him. It's a conversion symptom."

QUESTIONS:

1. What are conversion symptoms?

2. Name 10 commonly encountered conversion symptoms.

3. What distinguishes a conversion reaction from malinger-
    ing and from a psychophysiologic (psychosomatic) dis-
    order?

4. What is the relationship between conversion disorder
    and histrionic personality disorder?

5. Would hypnosis or a sodium amytal interview have any
    place in the diagnosis or treatment?

6. What type of personality does Edward appear to have?

7. What term refers to the hysterical inability to stand
    and walk?

ANSWERS:

1.   Conversion symptoms are motor or sensory phenomena
      which suggest physical (often neurological) disorders
      but which have psychological roots. They may occasion-
      ally represent symbolic expressions of the patient's
      psychological conflict. Edward's conflicts likely
      involve issues of independence and fear of abandonment.
      His dramatic symptoms seem to communicate anger and
      helplessness, provide attention and sympathy, and seek
      to restore his dependent position.

2.   The most common conversion symptoms are those that
      mimic neurological disease - paralysis, weakness,
      seizures, incoordination, aphonia, blindness, anosmia,
      anesthesia, paresthesia, tunnel vision, dyskinesia and
      akinesia. Others include vomiting, pseudocyesis
      (false pregnancy), and trouble swallowing (globus
      hystericus).

3.   "Malingering" implies that a person has conscious and
      voluntary control of the symptom(s) and that his
      deceptive illness behavior is undertaken in pursuit of
      some recognizable goal. The goal is commonly material
      reward (disability payments), avoidance of undesirable
      responsibilities, food and shelter (through hospital-
      ization), or drugs.
          Psychophysiologic disorders (such as asthma and
      peptic ulcer disease) show demonstrable physiologic or
      anatomic pathology. Emotional factors likely play a
      role as do genetics and environment. Also, psycho-
      physiologic disorders relate to the autonomic nervous
      system, rather than the voluntary sensorimotor system,
      and have no unconscious symbolic meaning (some would
      dispute these distinctions).

4.   Histrionic personality traits are common in those with
      conversion symptoms but are not always present. Modern
      studies show the concurrence rate to be about 50%.
      Histrionic personality traits - such as dependency,
      dramatics, attention-seeking, egocentricity, and man-
      ipulation - obviously provide a fertile setting for
      initiating and maintaining conversion symptoms.

5.   Probably. At least they would not likely be harmful.
      The diagnosis often becomes more obvious when, in an
      altered state of consciousness, the patient clearly
      reveals the conflict underlying the symptom or talks
      openly about his secondary gains. Also, with sugges-
      tion, the symptoms may totally remit.

An amytal interview was performed on Edward. During it, he cried continuously and emphasized his fear of independence, abandonment, and loss of love. His words, "I can't stand on my own," may be suggestive of the symbolic conflict.

6. Dependent personality (DSM-III, 301.60). Factors that appear to predispose one to conversion symptoms are dependent personality, histrionic personality, extreme psychosocial stress, exposure to other individuals with illness (either organic or conversion), and an antecedent physical disease (providing a model for symptoms).

7. Astasia-abasia.

PEARLS:

1. Conversion disorder is less common now than several decades ago.

2. The usual age at onset is adolescence or young adulthood; however, neither children nor the elderly are immune.

3. Most conversion symptoms remit spontaneously.

4. Most patients whose conversion symptoms remit do not show "symptom substitution" (where other symptoms quickly take their place).

5. Conversion symptoms that do not remit fairly quickly are more likely to be associated with massive secondary gain or undiagnosed organic illness.

6. Recurrent conversion symptoms most commonly occur in those with Briquet's disorder.

7. Some conversion disorders have been noted to come and go in response to life stresses.

PITFALLS:

1. Conversion symptoms are not limited to the unsophisticated and poorly educated patient. While dramatic or grossly nonphysiologic symptoms are most likely to occur in this group, more sophisticated patients have more sophisticated symptoms which closely approximate true medical disease.

2.   A symptom picture may be a mixture of physiologic and conversion symptoms - such as one with both "true" and "pseudo" seizures or one with unconscious exaggeration of bona fide medical symptoms. Don't identify <u>only</u> the conversion component of a complex picture.

3.   La belle indifference (a presentation suggesting relative indifference or unconcern for a severe symptom) is not as useful or consistent in conversion disorder as was once thought. It is present in a minority of such patients and is also found in the stoic medically ill and those with strong needs to deny the seriousness of their condition.

4.   Those with recognized histrionic personality traits are often dismissed outright from any serious medical attention. Such personality traits do not provide immunity from organic disease.

5.   Do not consider conversion disorder a "diagnosis of exclusion."

TRIVIA:

1.   Egyptian papyri dating back 4000 years describe diseases caused by a wandering uterus ("hysteria" - from the Greek word for uterus, "hustera"). Treatment consisted of various perfumes to attract the uterus back to its correct location.

2.   It is likely that many "witches" burned at the stake during the Middle Ages were actually hysterics presumed to be possessed by demons.

REFERENCES

1.   American Psychiatric Association Task Force on Nomenclature and Statistics: <u>Diagnostic and Statistical Manual of Mental Disorders</u>, 3rd ed. (DSM-III). Amer Psychiatric Association, Washington, DC, 1980.
2.   Ford CV: <u>The Somatizing Disorders: Illness as a Way of Life</u>. New York, Elsevier Biomedical, 1983.
3.   Hafeiz HB: Hysterical conversion: A prognostic study. Brit J Psychiat 136:548-551, 1980.
4.   Jones MM: Conversion reaction. Psychol Bull 87:427-441, 1980.
5.   Kaplan HI, Sadock BJ: <u>Comprehensive Textbook of Psychiatry</u>, 4th ed., Baltimore, Williams & Wilkins, 1985.
6.   Maloney JH: Diagnosing hysterical conversion reactions in children. J Pediatrics 97:1016-1020, 1980.

Index